Dementia Support for People from Diverse Ethnicities and their Families

of related interest

About University of Bradford Dementia Good Practice Guides

Under the editorship of Professor Murna Downs, this series constitutes a set of accessible, jargon-free, evidence-based good practice guides for all those involved in the care of people with dementia and their families. The series draws together a range of evidence including the experience of people with dementia and their families, practice wisdom, and research and scholarship to promote quality of life and quality of care.

Selected titles from the series

Human Rights in Dementia Care (August 2025)
A Good Practice Guide
Suzanne Cahill, Fiona Kelly and Helen Rochford-Brennan
ISBN 978 1 83997 063 4
eISBN 978 1 83997 064 1

The QCS Pool Activity Level (PAL) Instrument for Occupational Profiling
A Practical Resource for Carers of People with Cognitive Impairment Fifth Edition
Jackie Pool
ISBN 978 1 83997 502 8
eISBN 978 1 83997 503 5

LGBTQ+ People and Dementia
A Good Practice Guide
Sue Westwood and Elizabeth Price
ISBN 978 1 83997 330 7
eISBN 978 1 83997 331 4

DEMENTIA SUPPORT for PEOPLE from DIVERSE ETHNICITIES and THEIR FAMILIES

A Good Practice Guide

Jan Oyebode and
Sahdia Parveen

FOREWORD BY

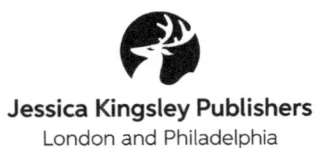

Jessica Kingsley Publishers
London and Philadelphia

First published in Great Britain in 2026 by Jessica Kingsley Publishers
An imprint of John Murray Press

Copyright © Jan Oyebode and Sahdia Parveen 2026

The right of Jan Oyebode and Sahdia Parveen to be identified as the Author of the Work has been asserted by them in accordance with the Copyright, Designs and Patents Act 1988.

Front cover image source: Shutterstock®. The cover image is for illustrative purposes only, and any person featuring is a model.

All rights reserved. No part of this publication may be reproduced, stored in a retrieval system, or transmitted, in any form or by any means without the prior written permission of the publisher, nor be otherwise circulated in any form of binding or cover other than that in which it is published and without a similar condition being imposed on the subsequent purchaser.

A CIP catalogue record for this title is available from the British Library and the Library of Congress

ISBN 978 1 78592 621 1
eISBN 978 1 78592 622 8

Printed and bound by CPI Group (UK) Ltd, Croydon, CR0 4YY

Jessica Kingsley Publishers' policy is to use papers that are natural, renewable and recyclable products and made from wood grown in sustainable forests. The logging and manufacturing processes are expected to conform to the environmental regulations of the country of origin.

Jessica Kingsley Publishers
Carmelite House
50 Victoria Embankment
London EC4Y 0DZ

www.jkp.com

John Murray Press
Part of Hodder & Stoughton Ltd
An Hachette Company

The authorised representative in the EEA is Hachette Ireland, 8 Castlecourt Centre, Dublin 15, D15 XTP3, Ireland (email: info@hbgi.ie)

Contents

1. Introduction and Overview. 9

2. Lifestyles and Risk of Dementia 15

3. Stigma and Awareness in Ethnic Minority
    Communities. 37

4. Being Diagnosed with Dementia 57

5. Living with Dementia in the Community 79

6. Using Care Homes 97

7. Advance Care Planning, End of Life and Bereavement . . 121

8. Conclusions. 145

   APPENDIX: MATCHING BEHAVIOUR CHANGE TECHNIQUES
   TO BARRIERS (MICHIE, 2011) 154

   REFERENCES 156

   SUBJECT INDEX 167

   AUTHOR INDEX. 174

TABLES

- **2.1:** Five layers of health determinants, based on Dahlgren and Whitehead's model (2021) 29
- **2.2:** Theoretical Domains Framework: 11 barriers to behaviour change with examples related to diet (Michie *et al.*, 2005) 33
- **2.3:** Strategies for Karina to overcome barriers to lunchtime exercise 34
- **2.4:** Top ten points for designing effective mass media health campaigns 36
- **3.1:** Key factors that influence perceptions of illness 46
- **3.2:** The Common Sense model of illness applied to the common cold 47
- **3.3:** A checklist for cultural adaptation of dementia awareness materials 55
- **4.1:** Barriers to the validity of cognitive assessments for minority ethnic populations 73
- **5.1:** Ten top tips for your cultural competency learning journey 96
- **6.1:** Examples of external pressures to continue to care at home 105
- **6.2:** Approaches to improving communication between staff and care home residents who do not speak fluent English 116
- **7.1:** Domains of the culturagram assessment framework (Goodorally, 2015) 137
- **7.2:** Key recommendations for health and care professionals formulating end-of-life care plans for people from minority ethnic communities 140

FIGURES

- **4.1:** A model for interventions to improve access to dementia assessment and services for people from ethnic minorities in the UK (reproduced from Kenning *et al.*, 2017) 68

ACTIVITIES

- **2.1:** How are you? 18
- **2.2:** Identify the risk factors 29
- **2.3:** Design your own social media campaign 37
- **3.1:** What do you think of when you think of dementia? 39
- **3.2:** Using the Common Sense model to think about dementia 48
- **3.3:** Design a dementia awareness information programme for the Nigerian community living in the UK 57
- **4.1:** Knowing the facts of assessment and diagnosis for minority ethnic groups 63
- **4.2:** Your plan for improving access to dementia assessment for people from minority ethnic communities 69
- **5.1:** Motivations for care 86
- **5.2:** Preparing for transition points 89
- **5.3:** Living well with dementia 90
- **6.1:** Identifying culturally suitable activities 113
- **6.2:** Identifying and acting on culturally related issues 119

OUR PERSPECTIVES AND PROJECTS

We bring complementary but overlapping approaches to thinking about ethnicity and dementia. Sahdia, as a health psychologist, has an interest in public health approaches and models of understanding. Jan, as a clinical psychologist, has an interest in family functioning and interventions. Prior to moving to the University of Bradford, we had both researched ethnicity and dementia (see, for example, La Fontaine *et al.*, 2007; Parveen, Morrison & Robinson, 2011). Since 2013, we have undertaken work together, including evaluating the Alzheimer's Society's Information Programme for South Asian Families (IPSAF) affected by dementia (Blakey, Parveen & Oyebode, 2016; Parveen, Blakey & Oyebode, 2018) and running and evaluating culturally adapted dementia awareness workshops for a range of ethnicities in Bradford (Parveen, Peltier & Oyebode, 2017). The Caregiving HOPE project, funded through Sahdia's Alzheimer's Society fellowship (2016–2018), explored current and future carers' sense of obligation, willingness and preparedness to provide care, comparing majority and South Asian carers. In the chapters of the book, we draw on data from this fellowship as well as, with her permission, interviews by Divya Chadha, one of Jan's previous students. More recently, we have jointly supervised three doctorate (PhD) students and we also quote their work. They and their projects are:

- Oladayo Bifarin (2022): *Intersections between culture, sociodemographic change and caring: A qualitative study of current and prospective family caregivers in mainland China.*
- Mohammed Akhlak Rauf (2023): *Optimization of care transitions: Understanding coping strategies of South Asian family carers of a relative with advanced dementia.*
- Saba Shafiq (2024): *Using the self-regulatory model to explore cultural understandings of dementia and inform a culturally sensitive intervention.*

We would like to acknowledge their work and thank them for giving us permission to use anonymized quotes from the interviews they conducted with people of Chinese, South Asian, Irish and Caribbean ethnicity.

In addition, we have referenced work by Sahdia and Professor Richard Cheston, who jointly led a programme of research funded by the National Institute for Health and Care Research (NIHR) to develop a South Asian Dementia Pathway that includes an online toolkit of culturally appropriate assessments and interventions (see: https://raceequalityfoundation.org.uk/adapt) and finally, we also drew on Sahdia's DEM-SAFE project, which is focused on co-designing public health interventions to improve brain health and reduce the risk of dementia in South Asian and African and Caribbean communities in the UK, also funded by the NIHR.

Sahdia Parveen, Associate Professor, Centre for Applied Dementia Studies, University of Bradford

Jan Oyebode, Professor of Dementia Care, Centre for Applied Dementia Studies, University of Bradford

Chapter 1

Introduction and Overview

Introduction

This short chapter provides an introduction and overview of *Dementia Support for People from Diverse Ethnicities and their Families*. Modern British society includes people who have come here from many parts of the world, bringing their own traditions, and often their own languages and religions. This gives us a wonderfully diverse range of ethnicities but also poses challenges for providing appropriate care and support. Health and social care professionals may feel inadequate and unprepared to provide culturally sensitive care. Our aim in writing this book has been to draw together research-based and experience-based knowledge about the ways that being from a minority ethnic group impacts on experiences of dementia and to highlight what sort of support is needed or beneficial. We hope the book will be an accessible source for busy practitioners who want a guide to evidence-based practice in their work with people from minority ethnic communities who have been diagnosed with dementia, and their families.

This chapter gives a brief introduction to ethnicity in relation to dementia care. We start by introducing the significance of ethnicity in dementia care, define ethnicity and outline issues around terminology. We go on to describe the main minority ethnic groups in the UK and summarize the numbers who are likely to be living with dementia. We then introduce ourselves and some of the research studies we will be drawing on in the body of the book, before providing an overview of the structure and content of the following chapters.

Dementia and ethnicity

Dementia is an umbrella term for a group of conditions estimated to affect about 800,000 people currently living in the UK. The dementias are strongly associated with age. They affect brain function, get progressively worse over time, and there are currently no curative treatments. Most people with dementia live with the condition for around seven to ten years (Todd *et al.*, 2013). Most of this time is spent living in the community. As people's functioning gets worse and they need more help, the majority of support usually comes from families. Services are necessary too, of course, to provide a diagnosis, to offer relevant information and advice, to provide interventions to address cognitive, emotional and behavioural issues, to put people in touch with peers, to help with personal care or social care as needed, to provide options if the person and family are struggling to manage, and to assist at end of life.

It is widely accepted that each person with dementia is unique and that care and support need to be person-centred to be helpful. This principle is enshrined in UK dementia guidance and policy. It prompts us to consider each person in the context not only of the challenges caused by dementia itself, but also in relation to their wider health, abilities, personality and life experiences, their sense of self and identity, their relationships with family and friends and the resources they have available to help them adjust, adapt and manage. Yet, ethnicity (a definition follows later), a dimension that is fundamental to every person's life, is often not put forward as a fundamental area for consideration.

People who are from the majority group in society may not often consider their ethnicity. It is taken for granted. We take it for granted that there is an obvious 'right way' to approach things because we have grown up and been socialized into a particular society and most people around us share our assumptions. It is often only when others, for example from minority ethnic groups, think and behave differently, that our taken-for-granted worldview is revealed to us. However, ethnicity is pervasive. It influences our values and beliefs, including the way we perceive dementia and what those with dementia and their family members tell others about it. It influences whether we are likely to seek help from a doctor, and when. It impacts on whether we trust professionals, feel their advice applies to us and whether we follow that advice. It affects whether we have a sense of duty or obligation to care, as well as who in the family provides care.

Inevitably, most dementia services, whether in the healthcare, social care or voluntary sectors, are set up around the needs of the majority of people affected: that is, older, English-speaking people, predominantly women, who have grown up and lived their lives in the UK. The evidence, which we present in this book, is that these mainstream services are not good at meeting the needs of most people from minority ethnic communities in the UK, resulting in a major area of inequity in dementia care. On the other hand, there is increasing knowledge about how to meet the needs of different minority ethnic communities and we hope this book conveys positive messages about how to take effective action.

Terminology

In this section we introduce the terms we use to refer to the groups of people who are at the heart of our book. Understandably, this is a sensitive and contested area (Aspinall, 2020; Ryder *et al.*, 2021). We have chosen to refer to 'ethnic minorities' or 'minority ethnic' communities and 'the majority population' or 'White British majority'.

'Ethnicity' refers to a group of people who identify with each other on the basis of perceived shared attributes that distinguish them from other groups. Those attributes may include shared ancestry, history, traditions, culture, language, religion, and so on (Lu *et al.*, 2022). Ethnic groupings may be broad or specific; for example, the Nigerian side of Jan's (co-author of this book) family could describe themselves as West African, Yoruba, or Ekiti. Broader groupings contain a great deal of variation and may become so broad that those included have very little in common, as with the Black category in the UK Census, which includes Black, Black British, Caribbean or African Black. Specific groups also include individual variation. When considering dementia care and its intersection with minority ethnic issues, it is important to think about the meaningfulness of the ethnic groupings we use.

It is usually recommended that ethnicity should be self-defined, as it involves our own view of ourselves (Lam *et al.*, 2023). However, the term 'minoritized communities', which refers to the marginalization of some groups by the majority population, can also be useful when thinking about issues of prejudice. In terms of self-definition, we have choice. Sahdia (co-author of this book), for example, could choose to describe her ethnicity as Asian British, Pakistani English, Yorkshire or a number of other descriptors, and Jan's options could include English, White English or Kentish, or we could both describe ourselves as British or European. Which label we use may depend on the context of where we are and who we are with.

Ethnicity is also a dynamic construct that may evolve over a person's lifetime and across generations. So, for example, older generations may be united by common values around family care which depend on having siblings or extended families available to care, but younger generations, who may have to relocate for work, or who may have smaller families, may be more accepting of a need for formal care services due to the shift in circumstances, or due to imbibing the more individualistic values found in the majority population.

Where referring to others' research or publications, we use terms they have used. These are often based on the UK Census categories. In the Census, the five high-level ethnicities are Asian or Asian British; Black, Black British, Caribbean or African Black; White; Mixed or Multiple ethnic groups; and other. Each of these ethnicities has sub-categories; for example, Asian or Asian British includes Bangladeshi, Chinese, Indian, Pakistani, other Asian. White British ethnicity is a sub-category of White that subsumes English, Welsh, Scottish and Northern Irish. The terms BME (Black and minority ethnic) or BAME (Black, Asian and minority ethnic groups) are also widely used in research. Terms are constantly evolving and shifting and an expression that is acceptable at one point in time or in one context may become devalued and pejorative (see Ryder *et al.*, 2021, for a critique of terms).

Ethnic minorities in the UK

Within the UK, White British ethnicity dominates, accounting for 79% of the population of England, 93% in Wales, 94% in Scotland and about 98% in Northern Ireland (Cuibus, 2024). Twenty-five per cent of the population of England and Wales classify themselves as being from one of the other ethnic groups, in other words as being from an 'ethnic minority'.

The composition of ethnic minorities in the UK has been shaped by empire and colonization (Shankley, Hannemann and Simpson, 2020). Substantial numbers of people came to the UK from colonies or former colonies, including the Caribbean and the Indian sub-continent, in the latter half of the 20th century, to fill the British need for labour after the Second World War. Others came or are coming to escape difficult conditions at home, such as famine and conflict. These include South Asian people who were expelled from East Africa in the 1960s and 1970s, and the Irish, who have a long history of movement from Ireland to the UK, to escape famine in the 1800s and more recently for reasons of work, lifestyle and education. These populations of Irish, Caribbean and South Asian descent are well established. They include generations born and bred in the UK and substantial numbers of older people. The ethnicities with the oldest population profiles are the Irish, followed by the White British, and the Caribbean population (Lievesley, 2013). Dementia is therefore most common in these communities. Current figures suggest that about 25,000 people from ethnic minority backgrounds have dementia. It is predicted that there will be a seven-fold increase in the number of people from minority ethnic communities living with dementia by 2050 (APPG: All Party Parliamentary Group on Dementia, 2013). The current century has brought new patterns of immigration, with more Chinese, African and Eastern European people moving to the UK (Shankley, Hannemann & Simpson, 2020; Cuibus, 2024). Although UK populations from these areas do not have very large older populations, they will in future, so it is relevant to think about needs now.

It should be noted that some parts of England and Wales are more ethnically diverse than others, with most diversity in London and the West Midlands and least in Wales and the

North-East of England (UK Government, 2024). This means that some dementia care services will need to cater for substantial minority ethnic communities, whereas other services may only occasionally meet ethnic minority families. These two scenarios pose different issues to address.

Content and structure of the book

This book is structured to follow the thread of living with dementia. We aim to show the influences of ethnicity at each step and the associated challenges these provide for people from ethnic minorities with a diagnosis, their families and care staff, along with possible ways to overcome those challenges.

To follow this thread, we have organized the chapters around the 'dementia journey'. The chapters cover prevention, awareness and stigma in communities, assessment and diagnosis, living with dementia in the community, making use of care homes and, finally, advance planning, end-of-life care and bereavement. Each chapter provides an account of key issues and support needs for people from minority ethnic groups, summarizing the evidence base and drawing on lived experiences. We include the voice of people living with dementia and their families, friends and carers to bring the issues to life. Each chapter is punctuated with activities and points for reflection or practice. In the final brief chapter, we bring together the key learning points across the book.

Chapter 2

Lifestyles and Risk of Dementia

Dementia is by no means an inevitable consequence of reaching retirement age, or even of entering the ninth decade. Lifestyle factors might reduce, or increase, an individual's risk of developing dementia. In some populations, dementia is already being delayed for years, while in others the number of people living with it has increased.

(LIVINGSTON ET AL., 2017)

Introduction

In this chapter, we summarize the evidence that suggests that some types of dementia are related to aspects of lifestyle that can be changed. These are known as 'modifiable risk factors'. We explore the key risk factors associated with dementia and look at how common these are in minority ethnic communities. We also consider what influences whether an individual is motivated and able to make lifestyle changes that could reduce their risk of developing dementia. By the end of this chapter, you should feel confident to talk with and provide information to minority ethnic communities about healthy living.

ACTIVITY 2.1: HOW ARE YOU?

Let's do a quiz!

If you scan the QR code, it will take you to Public Health England's 'How Are you?' quiz. The quiz will help you think about healthy lifestyles and key behaviours that lead to a healthier life.

You can also access the quiz using the following link: www.nhs.uk/better-health/how-are-you-quiz

Ethnic differences in dementia risk

Research on ethnic differences in dementia rates has produced mixed results. A systematic review of 19 studies found that people from South Asian or Black backgrounds were more likely to develop dementia compared to the White population (Shiekh *et al.*, 2021). However, the majority of the studies in Shiekh's review were American, and only two studies were conducted in the UK.

Mukadam *et al.* (2022) used data from a UK biobank to test ethnic differences and the impact of risk factors. A biobank is a collection of anonymized medical data from a large number of people. Mukadam included data from 294,162 people who had been followed up for almost 15 years. Mukadam reports that while African and Caribbean groups were more likely to develop dementia compared to White British groups, there was no difference between South Asian and White British groups. They also found the effect of dementia risk factors was the same across all ethnic groups. A further study explored ethnic differences using information from 1,016,277 primary care records collected in East London between 2009 and 2018 (Bothongo *et al.*, 2022). The study concluded that those from an African, Caribbean or South Asian background were more likely to develop dementia and at a younger age compared to the White British group. They found that ethnicity and the level of deprivation were better predictors of dementia risk than any modifiable risk factors.

While the findings that some ethnic groups may be at higher risk of dementia are interesting, ethnicity is not a risk factor that we can change. However, the emerging evidence that ethnicity may be a risk factor for dementia can help us prepare to be better able to meet the needs of certain communities. It may also prompt us to focus on enabling people in minority ethnic communities to address dementia risk factors that are more amenable to change through lifestyle modifications. In the next section, we present the modifiable risk factors associated with dementia.

Dementia and modifiable risk factors

In line with the idea that 'prevention is better than cure', there has been a growing amount of research focused on the risk factors associated with dementia. Although there are currently no treatments to cure dementia, it is thought that by targeting risk factors, there could be a delay in the onset of dementia. In fact, the current evidence on dementia risk factors suggests that a third of dementia cases may be preventable. Furthermore, there may be risk factors that are potentially reversible.

In 2017, Livingston *et al.* published an extensive review of current research evidence on prevention to produce recommendations on how to prevent and manage dementia (Livingston *et al.*, 2017). The review found that although numbers of people living with dementia may be declining in Western countries such as the UK, USA, Sweden, Canada and the Netherlands, the reverse is the case for Asian and African countries. The World Alzheimer Report (Prince *et al.*, 2015) predicted that 140 million people living with dementia in the year 2050 will be residing in low- and middle-income countries, compared to approximately 30 million people in high-income countries. Livingstone *et al.*'s review suggests that up to 35% of dementia cases result from lifestyle factors such as education, physical activity and cardiovascular diseases. The review presents the risk factors in accordance with when in the lifespan they are most relevant, from early childhood to later life. We will consider each risk factor below and the specific effects of each factor. It is worth noting that Livingston *et al.*'s review focused on evidence from high-income countries as there was little research from low- and middle-income countries.

Education

The level of education an individual has in their early life is the second most significant influence on the likelihood of developing dementia in later life (with hearing loss being the first most significant factor, see below). Research suggests that low levels of education – that is, primary school only – increases the individual's vulnerability to cognitive decline, because the individual has limited *cognitive reserve*. Cognitive reserve is when an individual develops spare (reserve) capacity for thinking, which gives them resilience to ageing and brain diseases. Those with higher levels of education tend to have higher levels of cognitive reserve. Cognitive reserve allows the individual to maintain intact day-to-day functioning despite brain changes. Ensuring that an individual has completed at least secondary school level education reduces the risk of developing dementia is by 8%. It is not known if education beyond secondary school level is of any further benefit to reducing the risk of developing dementia.

Hearing loss

There is a growing amount of evidence to suggest that even mild levels of hearing loss between the age of 45 and 65 years can increase the risk of developing dementia. Hearing loss may increase the risk of developing dementia by up to 9%. Why there is a link between hearing loss and cognitive decline remains unclear; it may be that hearing loss leads to people becoming isolated or depressed. A second theory is that hearing loss places extra strain on a vulnerable brain, thus increasing the risk of developing dementia.

Physical activity

Despite the positive effects of physical exercise, no research study has found that exercise prevents dementia. The current evidence base suggests that people aged over 65 years who are regularly physically active are more likely to maintain their cognitive functioning. There is some evidence that high levels of physical activity may have a protective effect and improve balance, mood and reduce falls, with physical activity in later life reducing the risk of developing dementia by 3% (Livingston *et al.*, 2017).

Diabetes/hypertension and obesity

There is evidence to suggest that hypertension (high blood pressure) and obesity in midlife (45–65 years) increase the risk of developing dementia by 3%. Obesity also increases the risk of developing diabetes, and diabetes in those over 65 years increases the risk of developing dementia by a further 1%. This may be because increases in inflammation and blood glucose impair an individual's cognitive abilities.

Smoking

Smoking in later life (over age 65 years) increases an individual's risk of developing dementia by 5%. This is because smoking is linked to various cardiovascular problems which impair an individual's cognitive abilities. It is also thought that the neurotoxins produced by smoking tobacco further heighten an individual's risk of developing dementia.

Depression

Depression in later life (above 65 years) is estimated to increase an individual's risk of developing dementia by 4%. There is some debate about whether depression is a symptom of dementia or a risk factor for its development. There is some evidence to suggest that depression increases the production of stress hormones, which in turn affect a person's cognition.

Social contact

Social isolation in later life is thought to increase an individual's risk of developing dementia by 2%. Current evidence suggests that social isolation increases the risk of hypertension, heart disease and depression. A lack of social contact in later life may also result in cognitive inactivity, which is linked to cognitive decline and low mood. As hypertension, heart disease and depression are risk factors for dementia itself, it is very important to consider the levels of social engagement of older people as well as their physical and mental health.

Other factors

Livingston *et al.* refreshed their original review of dementia risk factors in 2020 (Livingston *et al.*, 2020). They included three more risk factors in their life course model based on emerging evidence. They proposed that consuming more than 21 units of alcohol per week (equivalent to about 10 pints of beer, 9 medium glasses of wine or 21 shots of spirits) increased an individual's risk of developing dementia by 1% in midlife. Heavy drinking is also thought to be more associated with young onset (before the age of 65 years) dementia. Traumatic brain injuries (i.e. injuries from blows or knocks to the brain) experienced in midlife also added a further 3% risk of an individual developing dementia. Air pollution increased the risk of developing dementia by 2% in later life.

There is growing interest in identifying interventions than can reduce the risk factors associated with dementia and, at the same time, reduce the costs of services. Mukadam *et al.* reviewed potentially effective interventions and analysed their cost effectiveness (Mukadam *et al.*, 2020). They found that the most effective interventions were related to reducing diabetes and hearing loss, and smoking cessation. Interventions for reducing smoking and provision of hearing aids were found to be cost effective, and interventions related to hypertension prevention were cost effective in the UK only. Interventions for diabetes prevention were not considered cost effective. The authors concluded that if all three interventions (reducing hypertension, smoking cessation and hearing aid provision) were implemented, this would save England £1.863 billion per year and reduce dementia prevalence by 8.5%.

Modifiable risk factors and minority ethnic communities

Although there is evidence suggesting that people from minority ethnic backgrounds are more likely to develop dementia, a review of all the clinical trials related to dementia prevention found people from minority ethnic communities remained underrepresented in dementia research (Shaw *et al.*, 2022). Of 42 clinical trial reports they examined, just 26 reported ethnicity data and only 0.3% (i.e. 3 in every 1000) of participants were reported to be from minority ethnic backgrounds.

Despite the lack of people from minority ethnic backgrounds in dementia prevention clinical trials, there is growing evidence that certain risk factors may be more common in minority ethnic communities in the UK. In this section, we discuss the prevalence of lifestyle-related risk factors in minority ethnic communities and what types of interventions may reduce these risk factors.

Physical inactivity, obesity, hypertension and diabetes

Both diabetes and high blood pressure increase the risk of developing vascular dementia. Research suggests that those from South Asian backgrounds are less likely to take regular physical exercise and are more likely to have central fat distribution (fat around the stomach area), leading to higher levels of obesity (Oldroyd *et al.*, 2005). Obesity combined with nutritional factors such as low B12 and folate intake contribute to the development of insulin resistance and type 2 diabetes. It has been found that the rates of diabetes in the South Asian and the African Caribbean populations are four times higher than in the White British population (Wilkinson *et al.*, 2016). Wilkinson also found the onset of diabetes to be ten years earlier for individuals from a South Asian background than those from White British backgrounds. The progression of diabetes is much more rapid within the South Asian population and is also more likely to cause complications. While diabetes is much more common within the South Asian population, rates of hypertension are much higher among the African and Caribbean population in the UK. Oldroyd *et al.* found the incidence and prevalence of hypertension was much higher among the African Caribbean population (17%) with and without diabetes compared to the South Asian population (9%) and White British population (12%). The Chinese population had the lowest prevalence rates of diabetes, hypertension and heart disease in the UK.

Strategies to reduce blood pressure in minority ethnic communities have involved community screening, anti-hypertensive medication and education programmes focusing on salt reduction. However, as weight loss and physical activity can reduce the risk of hypertension and diabetes, the majority of interventions have focused on increasing physical activity. Despite the increasing number of interventions encouraging minority ethnic communities to exercise, South Asian and Black British communities remain the least physically active. An evidence review on barriers to exercising in South Asian communities (Patel *et al.*, 2017) found that although the communities had a good level of understanding regarding diabetes, they lacked knowledge about the level of exercise required for health benefits. There were a number of barriers to physical exercise, including: people prioritizing work over physical activity, different perceptions of 'ideal body weight' (being overweight was considered healthier and more attractive), and fear of racial abuse when exercising outside. Women experienced further barriers related to fear for personal safety, lack of same-gender spaces and concerns over the appropriateness of western exercise clothing. Similar barriers were found in a literature review focusing on Black British groups (Ige-Elegbede *et al.*, 2019). The authors reported that lack of knowledge of the link between physical exercise and health, religious/cultural expectations, social responsibilities and the lack of suitable environments to exercise were perceived barriers. The authors also noted the lack of research on Black British groups compared to South Asian groups.

Smoking

When people migrate to the UK, they often come from countries with very different legal frameworks for tobacco control (e.g. Eastern European countries) and different cultural approaches to tobacco use. According to the World Health Organization (WHO), countries such as Poland and Romania have much higher smoking rates (26% and 25.5% respectively) compared to 19.2% in the UK, whereas India, Pakistan, Jamaica and Nigeria (11.8%, 16.9%, 11%, 4.1%) have lower rates (World Health Organization, 2024a).

According to the UK Annual Population Survey (Office for National Statistics, 2024), the percentage of adults smoking cigarettes is much higher in White British groups (12.7%) compared to Black British (4.7%) and South Asian (7.4%) groups. There has been a steady decline in smoking rates in the UK across all ethnic groups. However, there is growing evidence that use of smokeless tobacco (tobacco products that are chewed, inhaled/sniffed, or placed in the mouth) is significant among minority ethnic groups. Action on Smoking and Health (2024) reported that 23% of South Asians reported using smokeless tobacco compared to 19% of Black/African/Caribbean groups and 12% of White British people. Smokeless tobacco use was highest in Bangladeshi men. A report from the National Institute of Clinical Excellence (NICE, 2021, updated 2023) emphasizes the need to reduce smokeless tobacco use in some South Asian communities, stressing the importance of working with communities to design and deliver support. Shisha pipes were also more commonly used among South Asian groups, where 15% used shisha more than once a year, compared with 8% of Black/African/Caribbean groups and 2% of White British people.

Although fewer people of South Asian and Black African or Caribbean ethnicities smoke, there is considerable evidence that minority ethnic groups are more susceptible to smoking-related illnesses such as cancer, diabetes and stroke. Interventions to reduce smoking in the UK have focused on education, legal regulation of tobacco products, reducing exposure to second-hand smoke, and nicotine replacement therapy.

Depression

There is a higher prevalence of later life depression in minority ethnic groups compared to White British groups (Williams *et al.*, 2015). Williams *et al.* (2015) predicted the prevalence of depression to be 15.5% for South Asian older adults, 17.7% for Black Caribbean older adults and 9.7% for White British older adults. In addition, in minority ethnic groups, depression, similarly to dementia (see Chapter 4), is less likely to be diagnosed; people are less likely to be prescribed medication and experience poorer outcomes. For example, it has been found that African Caribbean groups more frequently present with depressive symptoms but are less likely to be prescribed anti-depressants (Mansour *et al.*, 2020).

The barriers to accessing mental health services for minority ethnic communities are well documented and are similar to those around accessing dementia services. A review of 15 studies on South Asian people's experiences of using mental health services (Prajapati & Liebling, 2022) reported that barriers included: mistrust of healthcare professionals due to previous experiences of racism, services not being deemed culturally appropriate, and the desire to avoid the cultural stigma associated with mental health. Similar barriers have been identified to mental health service access in African Caribbean groups (Devonport *et al.*, 2023). Black British people were less likely to access services via a traditional pathway and were more likely to seek support from community leaders. Recently, there has been a 'push' to culturally adapt existing therapies for depression to ensure treatment is more culturally sensitive to minority ethnic communities. Cultural adaptations have included ethnic matching of therapists, language/translator provision, and incorporation of religious and cultural views within the therapy; for example, there has been work around religious adaptation of behaviour activation therapy for Muslim patients (Mir *et al.*, 2019). There is some evidence to suggest that culturally adapted therapies lead to better outcomes, but this is dependent on the level/depth of cultural adaptation (Rathod *et al.*, 2018). We explore this further in Chapter 3.

Lack of social contact

Loneliness has been linked to heart disease, stroke, depression, cognitive decline and early death (Valtorta *et al.*, 2018; Holt-Lunstad, 2020). Research suggests that older people from minority ethnic communities are more prone to loneliness, but the experience of loneliness differs across the different ethnic groups. Overall, it has been found that between a quarter and a half of older people from minority ethnic communities experience social isolation compared to one in ten White British people (Lewis & Cotterell, 2017). However, among mid-life and older people in the UK, it has been found that there is no difference between rates of loneliness reported by those of Indian ethnicity and the general population.

There are a number of factors that may lead to social isolation among minority ethnic groups, but the following are considered the most significant:

1. *Discrimination and racism*: This limits opportunities for social interaction.
2. *Social networks and community*: Due to various inequalities, minority ethnic communities are more likely to live in deprived neighbourhoods where there are fewer amenities and opportunities for social participation.
3. *Social and group identities*: Belonging to a particular group provides some protection against social isolation. Religious activities often provide important opportunities for social engagement.
4. *Health inequalities*: Factors that impact health and social quality of life are unequally distributed across minority ethnic groups. We discuss this further later in the chapter.

The number of older people living alone is likely to increase, resulting in higher levels of social isolation (Holt-Lunstad, 2020). Various national anti-loneliness campaigns have been developed to address this, for example by Age UK (n.d.). Strategies to reduce loneliness in older people have focused on increasing social contact via helplines, befriending services, lunch clubs, day centres, and social community activities. One review found that the most effective strategies to reduce loneliness were community-based art programmes, and technological solutions, for example online group activities, were also promising (Poscia *et al.*, 2018). Despite this work to combat loneliness, there is little evidence with regard to the impact on minority ethnic communities. It is likely that minority ethnic communities experience similar barriers to accessing these support programmes as they do in accessing health services.

In summary, a number of risk factors for dementia are prevalent in minority ethnic communities. These risk factors can be reduced via lifestyle changes: diet, physical exercise, social contact and smoking cessation. The majority of interventions aimed at influencing lifestyle change have focused on education without consideration for wider barriers to people implementing lifestyle changes (we refer to this as behaviour change). Before we consider how to help people achieve behaviour change, we need to understand the broader challenges people face in living a healthy life. In the next section, we explore health inequities and models used to explain what contributes to health inequalities.

The broader context of health

Social and economic factors or circumstances influence a person's ability to live healthily. These factors are also known as social determinants, that is, non-medical factors that influence a person's health. Social determinants are the circumstances that a person is born into, grows up in, works in, and grows older in. Some examples are income, education and housing conditions. According to the World Health Organization (2024b), social determinants account for 35–55% of health outcomes and can impact on health equity in positive and negative ways. They are important to consider in the context of health promotion and are considered an important influence on health inequities.

Health inequities and health inequalities

Although the terms 'health inequities' and 'health inequalities' are often used interchangeably, one is broader than the other. The National Institute of Clinical Excellence (NICE, 2024) defines health inequalities as 'differences in health across the population, and between different groups in society, that are systematic, unfair and avoidable'. The term 'health inequity' also refers to differences in health between groups but can also include differences in access to health services and the quality of care.

Over 30 years ago, Dahlgren and Whitehead presented a model summarizing the main social and economic circumstances that determine the health of a person or a community, which still stands today (Dahlgren & Whitehead, 2021). The model outlines five different layers of determinants, all of which need to be tackled to address health inequalities.

Table 2.1: Five layers of health determinants, based on Dahlgren and Whitehead's model (2021)

Number	Layer	Details
1	Individual characteristics	Including ethnicity, gender, age and hereditary factors
2	Individual lifestyle factors	Behaviours such as smoking, drinking and physical exercise
3	Social and community networks	Including family and wider social support
4	Living and working conditions	Access to health services, employment, housing, welfare, education, clean water and healthy food
5	General socio-economic, cultural and environmental conditions	The political climate, the strength of the economy, the availability of employment and disposable income

As health and social care practitioners, we are perhaps most able to influence layers 2, 3 and 4. In the next section, we consider how to delay the onset of dementia risk factors through lifestyle changes.

Lifestyle changes to delay the onset of dementia

We have outlined the main risk factors associated with dementia and identified which are more prevalent in minority ethnic communities. In this section of the chapter, we consider changes an individual can make to their lifestyle to reduce the risk of dementia.

ACTIVITY 2.2: IDENTIFY THE RISK FACTORS

The following table presents a number of case studies. Can you identify the corresponding risk factors? As a health and social care practitioner what suggestions can you make with regard to lifestyle changes which may help reduce the onset of dementia?

Case study	Risk factors	What lifestyle change would you suggest?	What is the level of difficulty to make this change?
Samara is a 50-year-old Pakistani working as a school administrator. She has noticed she cannot hear very well when people speak to her.			
Tierna is a 75-year-old Irish widow living alone at home. She can often go for weeks without speaking to a person.			
Hassan is a 35-year-old Indian man who has smoked since the age of 13 years. He was recently informed by his GP he is also pre-diabetic.			

Fiona is a 55-year-old from Ghana. She attended school up until the age of nine years. Since moving to the UK she has been suffering from depression.			
Naz is a 45-year-old Bangladeshi man. He has recently gained some weight and his blood pressure has been quite high for some time now.			

As health and social care practitioners we are ideally placed to influence lifestyle changes and promote behaviour change within the communities we work with. In the next section, we take you through an evidence-based approach to behaviour change in individuals and communities.

Achieving behaviour change

Lifestyles are made up of a range of health-related behaviours that are developed over time and influenced by our beliefs, abilities, attitudes and access to resources. Professor Susan Michie and colleagues (2005) proposed a theory of behaviour change known as the Theoretical Domains Framework (TDF). This is an evidence-based, easy-to-use model to guide effective behaviour change. Several versions have been created for use in different settings (e.g., hospitals vs community). The version that we present below combines elements of behaviour change with principles of implementation science (this addresses how to bring about changes that are likely to be adopted and maintained). It has four stages.

STAGE 1: IDENTIFY THE BEHAVIOUR

Choosing a behaviour to change appears simple but is more complex than it appears. The behaviour that is selected for change should be the most likely to have an impact on health. Let's consider the following example:

- Karina is a foodie and eats quite healthily. However, she has noticed that she has gained weight recently. She has an office job and sits at her desk for long periods of time.

What behaviour should she change? There are two obvious choices: she could eat less (restrict her diet) or exercise more. Karina already has a healthy diet so restricting calories may not help but she doesn't appear to exercise very much so may benefit from more physical activities.

In addition to identifying the behaviour most likely to have an impact, the behaviour needs to be SMART (specific, measurable, achievable, relevant and time bound).

- Karina will use her lunch break to do a 30-minute power walk, three times a week.

We have now identified a behaviour that is specific, measurable, achievable, relevant and time bound.

STAGE 2: IDENTIFY THE BARRIERS TO BEHAVIOUR CHANGE
In this stage, the goal is to find out what might prevent the person making the behaviour changes identified in stage 1. The TDF identifies 11 barriers that may stop a person changing their behaviour. We have outlined these in Table 2.2. If you can address the top three barriers to the person's behaviour change, you are more likely to achieve and maintain the behaviour change.

Table 2.2: Theoretical Domains Framework:
11 barriers to behaviour change with examples
related to diet (Michie et al., 2005)

Barrier	Meaning
Knowledge	Does the person know what a healthy diet consists of?
Skills	Does the person know how to cook a healthy meal?
Belief about capabilities	Does the person feel confident enough in their abilities to cook nutritious meals?
Motivations	Is the person motivated to cook a healthy meal?
Environment	Does the person have access to a kitchen to cook a healthy meal? Is healthy food available to the person?
Beliefs about consequences	Does the person believe that eating a healthy meal is a good thing?
Emotion	Does eating junk food make the person happier?
Social influences	Is the person around others who eat junk food?
Role/identity	How important is being seen to eat healthily to that person's sense of identity? Do they want to be a good role model?
Memory	Are they able to remember to eat healthy foods?
Action planning	Has the person planned how they will adopt a healthier diet?

You can work out what the barriers are for a person by discussing with them what might prevent them from doing the behaviour. Using the example presented above, you speak to Karina and identify the following barriers that might prevent her from her lunchtime power walks.

1. Related to motivation: Karina won't want to go out for a walk if it is raining.
2. Related to environment: Karina's colleagues eat lunch at their desks. She is worried about being the odd one out.
3. Related to action planning: Karina wears heels to work and won't remember to take flat shoes to work on walk days.

STAGE 3: MATCH BARRIERS TO BEHAVIOUR CHANGE TECHNIQUES
Michie and colleagues have produced a list of evidence-based behaviour change techniques that can be used to address the barriers described above (Michie, van Stralen & West, 2011). (You can see the behaviour change techniques that can be used to address each barrier in the Appendix at the end of the book.) Drawing on these, you can design practical strategies (or interventions) to help with behaviour change. We have drawn on these in Table 2.3, where we show ideas for how Karina can overcome barriers to achieving her exercise goal.

Table 2.3: Strategies for Karina to overcome barriers to lunchtime exercise

Barrier	Behaviour change technique	Practical strategy
Motivation	Practical problem solving	If it's raining, Karina could take an umbrella. Wear appropriate outerwear? Could she do her walk inside the building?
Social influence	Prompt identification as a role model	Karina could be a role model for her colleagues. She could ask them to join her and set up a lunchtime walking club.
Action planning	Use of prompts/memory cues	Karina will set a reminder on her phone to take flat shoes on her walking days. She could also leave flat shoes at work if permitted.

STAGE 4: EVALUATION AND MONITORING

Monitoring and evaluating the behaviour change is important to find out if the changes have been successful. There are two ways to evaluate the success of the behaviour change: process measures and outcome measures. Process measures are about whether an activity (or behaviour) has been completed. You could assess this by asking Karina to complete a diary or use an exercise app, so you can both track how often the activity was completed.

Outcome measures are about whether the health-related goal is achieved. Karina's goal is to lose weight. She will need to weigh herself before and after starting her power walks to see if she has lost weight.

It is important to consider process and outcome. If you only measure the outcome, and there has been no change, you may incorrectly conclude that the behaviour change technique you chose was ineffective. However, if Karina does not lose weight, it may have been that she never went out for the intended power walks. You cannot find this out without tracking process. If the process measures show she did not go on her walks, you can return to stage 2 to reconsider other barriers that may be preventing her from going out at lunchtime.

In Karina's case, we have worked on behaviour change with one person. It is possible to design behaviour change programmes for families and communities. If working with a community we would suggest setting up a stakeholder group to identify the key behaviour to change. To identify barriers and design practical strategies, we would suggest conducting discussion groups with the stakeholders, or if you are working across a very large region, conducting a survey. Evaluations of community behaviour change programmes are more complex and require public health and research methodology expertise.

Principles of effective health communication

In the section above, we primarily focused on individual behaviour change. While this works, it would be impractical and financially costly to implement individually tailored programmes with large numbers of people. Approaches that target entire populations reach many more people at a lower cost but are less likely to have an individual impact. On the other hand, even if only a small proportion of people change lifestyle as a result, this could make a difference on a population level (e.g., it might increase the numbers of people who eat five portions of fruit and veg each day). The presumed cost effectiveness of population-level campaigns is attractive to policy-makers, however, there is limited evidence about whether they work.

The most common population-level initiatives are mass media campaigns. A review of whether mass media messages about physical exercise, diet, tobacco and alcohol consumption targeting minority ethnic adults reduced the risk of diseases found only six studies, all of which were conducted in the US (Mosdøl *et al.*, 2017). The authors concluded that there was not enough evidence to understand whether mass media interventions lead to behaviour change which then leads to an impact on health.

Although the effectiveness of mass media health campaigns remains unclear, there are a number of ways you can ensure the health information you design is effective in changing attitudes. We present the top ten points to consider in Table 2.4 below.

Table 2.4: Top ten points for designing effective mass media health campaigns

Number	Key question	
1	Who is your target audience?	Information targeted to a specific group will be more effective in changing attitudes than generic information.
2	What is the existing level of knowledge in your target audience?	You may need to educate people about the risk factors of dementia first, before you can present them with persuasive messages to change behaviours that will reduce its risk.
3	What is your main objective?	Consider whether you want to educate the community or motivate people to change a specific aspect of their behaviour.

4	How will you disseminate the information?	You could produce a leaflet or present on a local radio show.
5	How will you ensure the information is accessible?	Will you translate into the target audience language?
6	How will you make your information eye-catching?	Think about design features your message should include. Find relevant photos and graphics.
7	How will you personalize communication to your audience?	Can you use personal pronouns? Think about the appropriate tone to use.
8	How will you ensure that your language is clear?	Take care to avoid jargon, use an active voice and everyday language.
9	How will you involve the community in designing and disseminating the information?	Speaking directly to the target audience will help you understand their needs.
10	Are the information and examples you use culturally appropriate?	You can consult people in the community on their views.

ACTIVITY 2.3: DESIGN YOUR OWN SOCIAL MEDIA CAMPAIGN

You have been asked to design a social media campaign to encourage men aged 35–45 years to quit smoking. Thinking about effective communication, record a short video that can be shared on social media.

To produce the video, think about the following:

- *Involvement:* How would you involve men aged 35–45 years?
- *Objective:* What are you wanting to achieve? Do you have a call to action?
- *Content*: What would the key messages be?

- *Communication channels:* What social media channels would you use to communicate the messages? How can you encourage people to share more widely?)

Conclusion

This chapter has covered the key risk factors associated with dementia. Dementia risk reduction is a growing area of research but to date there has been very little with minority ethnic communities. It is vital that more work is done with minority ethnic communities, as, otherwise, rates of dementia are likely to increase due to the higher prevalence of risk factors associated with dementia in these communities. There is little evidence to suggest that mass media campaigns to raise awareness of dementia risk factors will be effective. However, there are individual-level strategies we can use to help people adopt healthier lifestyles and potentially delay the onset of dementia.

Chapter 3

Stigma and Awareness in Ethnic Minority Communities

When you talk about dementia...this is a White, old White people's disease, it's not seen as Black people have dementia.
(JAMAICAN MAN, AGED 45–54, IN UK
43 YEARS; BERWALD ET AL., 2016)

Introduction
This chapter explores perceptions of dementia among minority ethnic communities in the UK and the impact of lack of community awareness on families affected by dementia. We consider current approaches for raising awareness of dementia and improving dementia education in minority ethnic communities. Finally, we present practical strategies that can be used to design and deliver culturally sensitive dementia awareness initiatives in the community.

ACTIVITY 3.1: WHAT DO YOU THINK OF WHEN YOU THINK OF DEMENTIA?

Write down all the words you can think of off the top of your head when you hear the word dementia.

Reflection: were the words positive or negative?

The importance of dementia awareness

In 2024, Alzheimer's Disease International published a report summarizing the findings from a survey of over 40,000 people from across 166 countries (Alzheimer's Disease International, 2024). It revealed that 88% of people living with dementia had experienced discrimination, and just over a third of respondents in low- and middle-income countries said they would want to keep their dementia a secret.

Unfortunately, a substantial number of people living with dementia around the world experience social stigma (the disapproval of, and/or discrimination against, people with characteristics which distinguish them from others, such as living with dementia). Stigma is thought to be caused by lack of education and awareness of dementia in society and can have significant consequences. The perceived stigma associated with dementia can lead to people:

- hiding their symptoms
- not seeking a diagnosis in a timely manner
- not receiving the appropriate treatment and support
- becoming socially isolated
- ultimately experiencing a poor quality of life.

The stigma associated with dementia is a global concern. It is therefore not surprising that dementia awareness and education are key priorities across all 48 countries with a national dementia strategy. A key feature of the UK National Dementia Strategy (Department of Health and Social Care, 2009) was to raise awareness of dementia and remove the stigma that surrounds the condition. The 2012 Prime Minister's Challenge on Dementia further elaborated on this and focused on creating dementia-friendly communities 'that understood how to help others' (Department of Health and Social Care, 2012). By 2015, the Alzheimer's Society had created 1 million dementia friends and there were 82 dementia-friendly communities; by 2020, there were more than 3 million Dementia Friends and 412 dementia-friendly communities.

Between 2012 and 2015, diagnosis rates increased from 42%

to 59%, implying the success of the Dementia Friends campaign. Although the momentum was lost during the Covid-19 pandemic and these campaigns were not refreshed, there have been basic gains in raising awareness of dementia in the general population. However, across the same period, little changed for minority ethnic communities. Research has continued to report the lack of dementia awareness in minority ethnic communities and under-representation in dementia services (Johl *et al.*, 2016; Parveen, Peltier & Oyebode, 2017; Hossain *et al.*, 2020).

The experience of stigma associated with dementia may differ within and across minority ethnic communities due to their contrasting understanding of ageing and dementia compared to the 'White' majority in the UK. The early stages of dementia may not be seen as an illness, and symptoms such as memory loss may be considered a normal part of growing older. As the symptoms become more advanced, they may be interpreted as signs of mental illness, which is often hugely stigmatized in minority ethnic communities. In addition to the level of stigma, people in 'majority' and 'minority' communities in the UK may experience different associated layers of stigma. For example, White British people living with dementia experience a double jeopardy (disadvantage caused by two sources at the same time) due to old age being perceived negatively and dementia adding a second layer of stigma. However, in minority ethnic communities, old age is valued and the cultural value placed on 'respecting your elders' is important. Yet people living with dementia from minority ethnic communities experience multiple jeopardy due to the disadvantage of having a 'migrant' or 'ethnic' label, the disadvantage of often being from a lower social economic status and the additional stigma of dementia. The consequences of stigma also differ across cultures, with minority ethnic families reporting condemnation and discrimination from their own cultural group, leading to social isolation not only for the person living with dementia but for the wider family.

To be able to reduce the stigma associated with dementia in minority ethnic communities, we need to understand the cultural influences and beliefs surrounding dementia. The next section explores specific beliefs and attitudes towards dementia held by minority ethnic communities.

Cultural perspectives on dementia

Most research with minority ethnic communities has focused on public awareness and knowledge of dementia. Below we provide a summary of over 20 years' worth of research with the largest minority ethnic groups in the UK.

A summary of research conducted between 2005 and 2013 and focusing on dementia awareness in minority ethnic communities in the UK found eight studies, all based on interviews and discussion groups with specific ethnic groups in different regions of the UK (Johl et al., 2016). Of the eight studies, seven included people from South Asian backgrounds, four were with Black communities, one with Eastern European and one with Irish communities. A common belief across all the minority communities was that dementia was a normal part of ageing. Fear of discrimination from their own communities meant that people often hid the family member living with dementia from society and cut ties with the extended family and friends. Religious beliefs contributed to stigma, as it was often believed that dementia was a punishment from God. There were religiously specific views of dementia, for example Muslim participants interviewed believed that dementia was caused by evil spirits, but this view was not common in Hindu or Sikh families.

Another summary of research published between 1970 and 2014, specifically focusing on the South Asian community and their awareness of dementia, reported that South Asian participants perceived people living with dementia to have poor personal hygiene, and this was considered a source of shame and embarrassment (Poole, Harrison & Hill, 2021). Similar to Johl et al. (2016), they reported that religion contributed to the stigma associated with dementia and there was a fear of judgement from the community.

A review of research with Black, African and Caribbean families reported that there was a lack of awareness of dementia in these communities, with many believing that dementia was only experienced by 'White people', as they had not met anyone diagnosed with dementia from the same ethnic background as them (Roche et al., 2021). Religion was viewed positively as being a source of healing and strength. It is worth noting that the majority of the studies in these three reviews were conducted before 2014.

In 2016, we conducted a project to explore specific beliefs about dementia among British Indian, African and Caribbean, and Eastern European communities in Bradford (Parveen, Peltier & Oyebode, 2017). Our findings were a little different to those of previous studies. All communities viewed dementia as an illness and attributed memory loss to biological brain changes. Dementia was not considered to be a normal part of ageing but as being associated with older age (which is correct). People were able to outline some symptoms of dementia, such as memory loss and personality changes. There were some misconceptions about risk factors, such as a belief that medication for blood pressure causes dementia. However, people were generally aware of potential contributors to dementia, such as diabetes and lack of exercise. Religion continued to be of importance to all communities, often as a source of support as many were unable or unwilling to access dementia support services. This change in dementia awareness may have been the result of extensive dementia awareness work conducted between 2013 and 2016 in Bradford or it may be part of a shift across minority ethnic generations.

Although dementia awareness may be improving in minority ethnic communities, stigmatizing beliefs continue. Between 2020 and 2021, Saba Shafiq conducted interviews with Afro-Caribbean and Irish families affected by dementia in West Yorkshire, as part of her PhD, which we were supervising (Shafiq, 2024). We found that religion continued to play a stigmatizing role, with dementia being perceived as being a punishment from God.

> Dementia comes from the word demented, the Latin word demented, so that in itself has its own connotation of craziness and you're mad and you're this. Working in the Caribbean helped a lot with the stigma around dementia, like could it be black magic, could it be... I don't know, I went to a presentation once, this is how it is, to a church, the church wanted to do some workshops on dementia awareness. And I went in the church, there's about 30 people in the church, and one of them, I'll never forget this woman, said, 'Is it because the person who's suffering with dementia didn't believe in God or didn't go to church?' Now, I can imagine that being said for all the religions, whether they didn't

> go to the mosque, whether they didn't read the Koran or didn't go and read the...you know the religion part of it. *(Laura and Jade, African Caribbean carers, interviewed by Saba Shafiq, 2024)*

Our findings suggested that perceptions of dementia in the Irish community are similar to those of other minority ethnic communities, at least among the small number of people we interviewed. Dementia was not widely known, as families 'hid the person with dementia' due to feelings of shame and fear of judgement.

> Well, when I was in Ireland, I never met anyone with dementia. Well not that I know of. I actually think it was sort of kept, in their own family sort of thing. *(Niall, Irish person living with dementia; Shafiq, 2024, p.106)*

As with other communities, there was no specific word for dementia and it was referred to as 'memory problems'. The lack of a term for dementia has been seen as contributing to lack of awareness in a number of minority ethnic communities. Many dementia awareness initiatives have translated dementia as 'memory problems' to reduce the stigma and mental health connotations of dementia. However, the connotation has proved to be problematic (as has also been the case when this euphemism is used in English). We discuss this further below in 'Promoting dementia awareness and education'.

> I mean, I come from an Irish background. They don't even use the word dementia, they call it memory problems, you know, and it's you know, it's still a frowned upon kind of thing. *(Jack, Irish person living with dementia; Shafiq, 2024, p.86)*

While knowledge of dementia remains low in minority ethnic communities, families' responses to stigma from the wider community may be changing. Previous research presented by Johl *et al.* (2016) suggested that families from minority ethnic communities often hid the person living with dementia out of fear and shame, caused by the stigmatizing views of the wider community. We conducted interviews with South Asian carers living across the UK between 2016 and 2018 and were struck by their changing attitudes towards the wider community. Our more recent interviews with South Asian carers found that while carers were very aware of the stigma in the wider community, many no longer feared judgement.

> I don't really give a damn about what anyone else thinks. It's our life, we know what we're dealing with, we know how hard it is, we know how vulnerable she is, we understand the situation better. In our experience again we're finding that the Asian community is less understanding of the disease itself, anything mentally related, the Asian community in our experience tend to think you're a nut job. You've lost your marbles, you've gone doolally. So I'm finding in the Asian community there is a massive misguidance of different types of mental illnesses. They just tar everything with the same brush and everything is doolally. I don't really give a damn what anybody else thinks. *(South Asian daughter, caring for her mum living with young onset dementia; Caregiving HOPE study)*

This shift in attitudes may be fuelled by the younger generation, who are more educated and perhaps less inclined to follow cultural values.

The majority of the research to date has focused on South Asian and to some extent Black communities, and little is known about the experiences of Eastern European, Irish and other ethnic minority communities in the UK. While it is tempting to think in simplistic terms that certain ethnic groups have certain beliefs related to dementia, there is considerable variation within cultural groups (e.g., between South Asians) and considerable commonalities across cultural groups (e.g., between South Asian and White British). These differences are caused by levels of acculturation, education, age, gender, personality, and family influences. In the next section, we explore how people develop perceptions of dementia and how they are influenced.

Understanding perceptions of dementia

Dementia awareness is important because how we perceive and understand dementia influences whether we seek a diagnosis and support. But what shapes our understanding of an illness? Key factors influencing perceptions of dementia are shown in Table 3.1.

Table 3.1: Key factors that influence perceptions of illness

Factor	Specific influences
Culture	Western cultures tend to divide the mind, body and soul and take a biomedical approach to managing illness. In many other cultures, a more holistic approach is common and spiritual well-being is as important as physical well-being.
Gender	There is considerable research that suggests men are more likely to ignore their symptoms and less likely to access health services.
Age	Knowledge and perceptions of illness are often abstract. It is not until the age of 12 years that people develop an understanding of illness and can understand abstract ideas.
Personality	There is some evidence to suggest that people with more neurotic personality types (i.e., those who are born worriers) are more likely to notice their symptoms early and seek help.
Family	Families can also shape how you understand and perceive illnesses, for example you are more likely to ignore your symptoms if your family does not perceive your symptoms as serious.
Media	The media often creates negative stereotypes and stigma around illnesses, for example through the portrayal of characters on TV shows or the language used in newspapers ('demented' and 'suffering' are common terms used by journalists that people living with dementia have challenged).

The biggest influence on our understanding of illness is personal experience.

A common theory used in healthcare research to explore people's understanding of illness is the 'Common Sense model'

(Leventhal, Phillips & Burns, 2016), also known as the 'Self-Regulation' model. This suggests that how you perceive an illness will affect how you cope with it and whether you seek help. The model proposes that a person's perception of an illness has different aspects. Imagine that your brain stores information about different illnesses in folders; for example, what you know about dementia is kept in a separate folder from what you know about the common cold. Imagine that each folder contains several tabs where you can store information about different aspects and add new information over time. The updated 'Common Sense' model (Weinman *et al.*, 1996) suggests that information about any illness is stored under nine tabs: identity (signs and symptoms), cause of illness, consequences of the illness, timeline (how long it will last), illness coherence (a deeper understanding of the illness that goes beyond naming symptoms), cure, personal control (things you can do to help yourself, such as attending a dementia well-being cafe), treatment control (medical treatments that help manage the illness), and emotional representations (the emotional response to an illness).

To understand the model on a practical level, let us consider the common cold. Table 3.2 contains the different tabs that represent illness perceptions and the type of information that might be stored under each tab.

Table 3.2: The Common Sense model of illness applied to the common cold

Illness perception category	Definition	Information
Identity	Signs and symptoms	Sneezing, cough, fatigue
Cause	What caused the illness	Germs
Consequences	What are the consequences of the illness?	Have to miss work and stay inside
Timeline	How long will the illness last?	Three to seven days

cont.

Illness perception category	Definition	Information
Cure	Can the illness be cured?	No
Coherence	Deeper understanding of the illness	It's a minor common condition. Not the end of the world. Will rest for a couple of days then I will be fine
Personal control	Can I help myself? What can I do to help myself?	Drink warm drinks. Rest.
Treatment control	Is medical treatment needed? Will medication help?	Take paracetamol
Emotional representation	What emotional response will I have?	Feel grumpy

ACTIVITY 3.2: USING THE COMMON SENSE MODEL TO THINK ABOUT DEMENTIA

We asked a group of young people aged 13–16 years to list all the words that came to their mind when they heard the word 'dementia'. We present the most common 15 phrases below.

Memory problems	Old people	Disease
Depression	Lonely	Sad
Head injury	Personality changes	Terminal
Confused	Bad genes	Angry
Loss of independence	Get lost easily	Disorganized

Organize these perceptions of dementia into the 'tabs' of the Common Sense model:

Reflection:

- How did the list produced by the young people compare to the list you created at the start of this chapter?
- Were the young people's perceptions positive or negative?
- Were their perceptions accurate?
- Did you notice a lot of the words would be categorized under 'Identity'?
- What were the main gaps in their knowledge?

We noticed that while there was some awareness of the basic signs and symptoms, the young people knew very little about the experience of living with dementia and the diagnosis had very negative connotations. They also knew very little about 'personal control' and 'cause' but expressed an interest in finding out more. By understanding young people's specific perceptions of dementia, we were able to identify the gaps in their knowledge. This enabled us to develop a targeted educational workshop that improved and deepened their understanding. The workshop presented young people with videos of people living with dementia discussing their lives, what they enjoyed doing and what they now found difficult. The young people brainstormed activities that they could do with a grandparent living with dementia to enable them to live well with dementia. They also learned about personal risk of dementia and self-reflection activities to consider why a person living with dementia may experience negative emotions, for example becoming sad when their needs are not met.

In the next section, we explore dementia awareness and education initiatives that have been developed for minority ethnic communities and the impact these awareness campaigns have had on families affected by dementia and the wider communities.

Promoting dementia awareness and education

As mentioned earlier in this chapter, the most common programme to raise awareness of dementia in the UK is the Dementia Friends programme delivered by the Alzheimer's Society.

The programme has been reported to be a success in promoting social inclusion and positive attitudes in the public. However, there are very few published evaluations of the programmes. Most have focused on a specific group (e.g., healthcare students) or a particular geographical region. The evaluations suggest that attending a Dementia Friends session led to improved knowledge and some small changes in attitude for participants (Baillie, Beecraft & Woods, 2015; Mitchell *et al.*, 2017; Berning *et al.*, 2023). The Dementia Friends programme was adapted somewhat for minority ethnic communities as materials were translated into several languages; however, it is unknown if this had any positive impact on minority ethnic communities. A review of dementia-friendly initiatives suggested that although dementia-friendly communities promoted social inclusion for people living with dementia, people from minority ethnic communities were not very involved in these initiatives (Shannon, Bail & Neville, 2019).

Our interviews with South Asian carers in the Caregiving HOPE study, conducted between 2016 and 2018, suggest that Dementia Friends did have positive impact on some families. A number of the carers had attended a Dementia Friends session and spoke positively about it. They were aware that dementia was caused by 'a disease of the brain' and was an illness. The English Dementia Friends session emphasizes that dementia is not just memory loss. However, as there is no word for dementia in South Asian languages, 'dementia' had been translated to 'memory problems' in South Asian language versions. Therefore, memory and dementia became synonyms for South Asian carers. This was unproblematic in the early stages of Alzheimer's dementia, but carers were left confused and stressed as the dementia progressed and the person with dementia had more complex needs. These needs were often left unmet due to carers' lack of understanding of the advanced stages of dementia, resulting in the person with dementia often becoming angry and the family feeling stressed. The carers believed the person was 'acting out' and 'being difficult on purpose' and didn't associate advanced symptoms with dementia.

> **POINT FOR REFLECTION: TRANSLATING 'DEMENTIA' INTO 'MEMORY PROBLEMS'**
>
> Has translating 'dementia' into 'memory problems' been helpful for service providers and South Asian families? Consider the following:
>
> - In Chapter 2, we discussed that risk factors for vascular dementia are more common in minority ethnic communities. Symptoms include: confusion, trouble concentrating and reduced ability to organize thoughts and actions. But memory problems are a common symptom of Alzheimer's disease (another type of dementia).
> - Earlier in this chapter, we stated that the word 'dementia' has social stigma attached to it. Could using the phrase 'memory problems' be a way of reducing the stigma?

Another common approach to promoting dementia awareness has been translating leaflets into various languages for minority ethnic communities. Although this is a relatively cheap and easy way to communicate information to a community, it is not the most effective way of raising awareness of dementia in minority ethnic communities. Usually, non-English-speaking older family members are also unable to read or write in their first language. They often rely on younger family members to read information to them, yet younger family members usually can read English but not the 'mother tongue'. Therefore, translated leaflets may not be useful for families.

In 2020, as part of the ADAPT study (in collaboration with the universities of West England, Bath and Wolverhampton, and the Race Equality Foundation), we worked with South Asian families affected by dementia and workers from third-sector community support groups to culturally adapt the dementia care pathway. South Asian families expressed that they would prefer dementia awareness sessions to be conducted in face-to-face sessions at their local community groups, and be delivered by a bilingual facilitator in collaboration with a healthcare professional. They wanted the sessions to focus on signs and symptoms, how to support the person living with dementia and information related to prevention.

> Because you see, it's no good if somebody's been diagnosed and given loads of literature, that person is not going to read it. Because the diagnosis and the thought of having a diagnosis of a condition that has got no cure, his confidence, his concentration is well and truly gone. And he's not going to read the leaflets, he needs a face-to-face, or somebody actually sitting in front of me and explaining what it is that he's got and how to overcome it.
> *(South Asian male, living with dementia)*

> **POINT FOR PRACTICE: THE ADAPT TOOLKIT**
> Our research shows that people prefer culturally adapted resources. The ADAPT study led to the development of a toolkit of culturally adapted resources to raise awareness of dementia in South Asian communities. You can access the toolkit by scanning the QR code with your phone, or use the following link: https://raceequalityfoundation.org.uk/adapt.

Beyond leaflets, there have been a variety of dementia awareness initiatives across the UK for minority ethnic communities which emphasize that dementia is an illness, with biomedical causes that can affect anyone. These may help dispel stigma (Mukadam et al., 2011, 2015; Mukadam, Cooper & Livingston, 2013; Kenning et al., 2017).

> If people were introduced to the fact that there is a physical cause... I think if things are explained in a simple and logical manner, it'll become more approachable, and understandable, and acceptable. *(Mukadam et al., 2015, p.6)*

Few such initiatives have been formally reported or evaluated so their impact is unknown. Below we present three initiatives that have been evaluated with promising results.

The East-Dem project (Mukadam, Cooper & Livingston, 2018)

South Asian people registered at a GP surgery in London were given a DVD encouraging people to seek help for memory-related problems. Only 41% of the people who received the DVD watched it but those who did appeared to be more likely to seek help as a result.

The IDEMcare project (Roche et al., 2018)

This project involved sending a letter and a leaflet about dementia to Black patients registered at a London GP surgery. The researchers reported that almost 94% of people accepted the leaflet, and at least 79% stated that they read it. Approximately 67% said they would consider seeking help as a result of reading the leaflet, and four people booked appointments with their GP to discuss memory problems.

The IPSAF project (Parveen, Blakey & Oyebode, 2018)

The Information Programme for South Asian Families project (IPSAF) was created by culturally adapting an existing Alzheimer's Society information programme for carers of people living with dementia. The original programme was poorly attended by South Asian families, so the Alzheimer's Society worked with community organizations to adapt the programme to be more culturally appropriate for South Asian families. The programme was delivered by the Alzheimer's Society in collaboration with local community organizations across 15 regions of the UK. The four face-to-face sessions covered: Understanding dementia, Legal and financial aspects, Supporting the person with dementia, and Looking after yourself. We evaluated the programme and found that it improved knowledge and fostered a deeper understanding of dementia. This led to positive changes in care practices and enabled the person living with dementia to feel more empowered and independent. Families reported being more aware of services and expressed the intention to access support as a result of the programme.

In the next section, we present a practical checklist that you can use to adapt existing dementia awareness and education to be more culturally sensitive for the communities you are working with.

Culturally competent engagement with communities

As mentioned earlier, a common way of raising awareness of dementia in minority ethnic communities is by translating existing materials. To truly create culturally sensitive materials, a deeper, more meaningful adaptation is required. Below we present key areas to consider followed by a checklist to use when evaluating the cultural adaptation of your materials.

- *Mode (format) of delivery:* It is tempting to use a tried and tested method for sharing information, such as leaflets. However, as we have discussed above, leaflets are not always the most suitable method for non-English-speaking communities. You may need to consider other modes of delivery such as face-to-face sessions or a video.

- *Setting:* While it may be easier to deliver a session on dementia awareness in your place of work, consider if this is a place that people naturally visit and where they feel comfortable. The setting needs to be based on the preferences of the community, for example a local community centre or a place of worship.

- *Delivery:* Consider who will deliver the information and what expertise is needed. Also consider the languages the information needs to be available in. Trusted messengers could be a highly educated professional, such as a doctor, or a religious or community leader, depending on context and topic (Mukadam, Cooper & Livingston, 2013; Shafiq, 2024).

- *Content:* It is not enough to translate information, as meanings are often lost and examples may not be culturally relevant. For example, in the Dementia Friends sessions, a common example used to illustrate the complex stages involved in a day-to-day activity was 'making a cup of tea'. In some cultures, this example may be irrelevant as older people may not be involved in household activities, and it may even be disrespectful to suggest that an older person may make a cup of tea.

In our culture, my grandfather if he's retired, he's sitting in the room, he's not making his cup of tea! My child, his grandchildren, or I will make cup of tea, and I will take the teacup and go into the kitchen. So he doesn't know where the sugar is or where the tea bags are, so he doesn't realize that he is losing his memory. (South Asian interviewee; ADAPT study)

Culturally relevant examples are important. They also need to be conveyed using appropriate culturally relevant images so that those watching a video or attending a course see others with whom they can identify.

Table 3.3: A checklist for cultural adaptation of dementia awareness materials

Criteria	Notes	Your evaluation of whether the criterion is met			
		Yes	No	To some extent	Not relevant
Do the materials have a clear focus on the community you are working with?	Does the leaflet feature photos of the community? Do the promotional materials name the community?				
Is the material to be delivered by community workers from the same background?	Preferably bilingual workers.				

cont.

Criteria	Notes	Your evaluation of whether the criterion is met			
		Yes	No	To some extent	Not relevant
Are the materials available in the preferred community language?	What languages should the materials be translated into?				
Is the translation linguistically accessible?	Have the materials been translated into lay language?				
Is the setting/location of the programme accessible?	Is it a setting people can get to easily and feel comfortable in?				
Has the delivery mode been culturally adapted?	If you're raising awareness via radio, are you on a station and radio show that is listened to by your target community?				
Has the content of the message been culturally adapted?	You may need to consider faith, diet, migration history, family roles, and experiences of community.				
Do your materials demonstrate cultural understanding?	Have you included people from the community with lived experience as experts?				
Do you have specialist knowledge of dementia?	Do you need specialist input from health or social care professionals?				

Does the programme have an evidence base?	If you are adapting an existing dementia awareness programme, is there evidence to suggest it is effective with the majority or other populations?			

The above is not an exhaustive list but we hope it will help you consider the different aspects of culturally adapting materials to raise awareness of dementia in minority ethnic communities.

ACTIVITY 3.3: DESIGN A DEMENTIA AWARENESS INFORMATION PROGRAMME FOR THE NIGERIAN COMMUNITY LIVING IN THE UK

Things to consider:

- Nigeria has a diverse population of different ethnicities, religions and languages. Identify which communities you are trying to reach.
- What is the community understanding of dementia? How can you find out?
- Use the Common Sense model to map out the dementia perceptions in the Nigerian community. Are there any key misconceptions or gaps in the knowledge?
- What are your key messages you need to share with the Nigerian community?
- How will you deliver the information and in what setting?
- What resources and expertise will you need?
- How will you know if the project has been a success?

Conclusion

It is vital to reduce the stigma associated with dementia among minority ethnic communities. An effective method of reducing stigma is through awareness raising and educating communities about dementia. There has been considerable interest in exploring the perceptions of dementia held by minority ethnic communities in order to develop targeted and culturally sensitive dementia awareness initiatives. In this chapter, we have highlighted how perceptions of dementia are changing across communities and how to identify specific misconceptions using the Common Sense model. We have also presented a checklist to facilitate the adaptation of existing dementia education materials to be more culturally sensitive.

Chapter 4

Being Diagnosed with Dementia

You don't know what the hell's going on with your father...then afterwards when we got the diagnosis it was like, 'Wow, that's what it was.' And then you had something tangible to work with now.

(TWO BRITISH SISTERS OF AFRICAN-CARIBBEAN ETHNICITY, INTERVIEWED BY SABA SHAFIQ)

Introduction

In this chapter, we consider the process of dementia assessment and diagnosis for people from minority ethnic communities. It is widely assumed that diagnosis is helpful, to give an explanation for changes and enable future planning and access to services. As a result, within UK health policies, there has been a push to increase rates and timeliness of dementia diagnosis (Department of Health and Social Care, 2015). However, different dementia perceptions and care values, distrust of services, service shortcomings and stigma may deter people from minority ethnic communities from seeking assessment and diagnosis. In addition, some aspects of dementia assessment may not be suitable for people of different cultural backgrounds. Diagnosis may not carry the assumed benefits if stigma prevents discussion of advance care plans and services don't offer acceptable support. We start with some facts and figures addressing common myths around minority ethnic diagnosis. We then look at community and service-related barriers to seeking a diagnosis and how these can be addressed. Following this, we examine the process of assessment, including issues of language and interpretation, interviewing and history-taking, and cognitive and functional assessment.

Background statistics

There are many myths about dementia assessment and diagnosis in minority ethnic communities. In this first section, we outline information from some of the most thorough research studies in the UK that have sought to find out whether there are ethnic differences around dementia assessment and diagnosis. We have picked out key findings using bullet points.

Are minority ethnic people being referred for dementia assessment?

In the past, those working in dementia services reported that people from minority ethnic communities were not referred in the numbers expected. However, recent data suggests this situation has changed and those from minority ethnicities are being referred to services, at least in the London area, in the expected numbers.

One study looked at referrals across 19 London-based memory services (Cook *et al.*, 2019). The authors found that:

- six services received the number of referrals expected, nine had more and four had fewer than expected from minority ethnic communities
- for South Asian populations, 11 services had expected levels. When services had lower levels, the shortfall was, on average, just 5%
- for Black communities, 12 services had expected levels, with a maximum shortfall of 2% across the others.

This picture was also seen in another large London study (Mukadam *et al.*, 2019), in which numbers of Asian and Black people seen in memory assessment services were at about the level expected from the population figures.

This generally positive picture, however, hides variation. Cook *et al.* (2019) found lower referral rates for people from Chinese and Pakistani communities, and one study (Adelman *et al.*, 2011) found people of African-Caribbean descent were less likely to have been referred by their GP to specialist dementia assessment services than the White British. This difference was not statistically significant, meaning it may have occurred by chance, though it sounds large:

- Just over half (54%) of African-Caribbean people over 60 with cognitive impairment were referred to specialist services by their GP, whereas 86% of the White British were referred.

Do people from minority ethnic backgrounds approach services later than the White British?

Professionals commonly report that people with dementia from minority ethnic communities come to services later than those from a White British background. It is hard to establish whether this is genuinely the case or not.

The most thorough UK study to date (Mukadam *et al.*, 2019) looked at two large London NHS Trusts, covering a population of 1.8 million people, over an eight-year period. The researchers looked at numbers of dementia diagnoses and scores on the Mini Mental State Examination (MMSE; Folstein, Folstein & McHugh, 1975) in over 13,000 people. They found that:

- MMSE scores were significantly lower in Asian and Black groups than in the White British. The average scores were one to three points lower, depending on ethnicity and NHS Trust. When socio-economic deprivation was taken into account, the differences still remained.

Having poorer cognitive functioning at the point of diagnosis implies dementia is more advanced by the time it is diagnosed. However, many commonly used cognitive screening tests have limited cultural validity. So, we need to be cautious in concluding that people from minority ethnic communities come later to services. It may just be that the commonly used tests over-diagnose (see the section 'Cognitive screening and assessment' later in this chapter).

Are people from minority ethnic backgrounds more or less likely to be diagnosed with dementia than the White British?

It is a mixed picture. One 'big data' study looked at variation in diagnosis rates by ethnicity, across over two million primary care health records from 2007 to 2015 (Pham *et al.*, 2018). They found, compared with White women and men:

- Black women were 25% *more* likely to receive a new diagnosis of dementia
- Asian women were 18% *less* likely to receive a new diagnosis of dementia
- Black men were 28% *more* likely to receive a new diagnosis of dementia
- Asian men were 12% *less* likely to receive a new diagnosis
- of dementia.

Are people from minority ethnic communities more likely to have vascular dementia?

Current research evidence is that this is true for some minority ethnic groups but not others. A study of over 12,000 health records of people with dementia in London (Tsamakis *et al.*, 2021) compared the type of dementia diagnosis across people from White British, White Irish, White other, Black Caribbean, Black African and South Asian backgrounds. They found:

- Black Caribbean (39%), Black African (42.9%) and White Irish (34.8%) were more likely to be diagnosed with vascular dementia than the White British (27.8%)
- rates of vascular dementia for South Asian (27.2%) and White other (30.4%) did not differ significantly from the rates for the White British.

Do people from minority ethnic backgrounds get dementia earlier in life than people from White British backgrounds?

A figure commonly cited as indicating that young onset dementia is more common in minority ethnic populations is that 6% of people from minority ethnic communities experience young onset dementia compared with 2% overall (Dementia UK, 2007).

However, although people from minority ethnic backgrounds are younger on average at point of diagnosis than the White British, the differences are likely to reflect differing age profiles of populations rather than a higher propensity to develop young onset dementia in minority ethnic populations.

One study of two large mental health Trusts (Mukadam *et al.*, 2019) found:

- the average age of the White British was 82 years when diagnosed, whereas the average age for the Black British was 78–79 years and for the Asian sample was 77–78 years.

A smaller study focusing on the Black population in a London memory service found that the Black population were diagnosed on average 4.5 years younger than the White British (Tuerk & Sauer, 2015).

ACTIVITY 4.1: KNOWING THE FACTS OF ASSESSMENT AND DIAGNOSIS FOR MINORITY ETHNIC GROUPS

In this section, we have presented information to support, or not, some of the main headlines about ethnic differences in relation to dementia diagnosis. In light of the information shown above, consider how firmly you believe each of the statements below:

- People from minority ethnic groups are not referred to memory services.
- People from minority ethnic groups are less likely to be diagnosed with dementia than White British groups.
- Black ethnic groups are more likely to be diagnosed with dementia than White British.
- South Asian groups are more likely to be diagnosed with dementia than White British.
- People from minority ethnic groups are more likely to be diagnosed with vascular dementia than White British groups.
- People from minority ethnic groups are diagnosed at a younger average age than the White British.

- People from minority ethnic groups get their diagnosis at a later stage of dementia than White British people.

You may have found you could not often answer with a simple yes or no. The research shows a complex picture, which reinforces that we cannot generalize across or even within minority ethnic groups. It also shows that ethnicity does not stand alone but 'intersects' with other individual characteristics, such as gender, and societal characteristics such as the degree of diversity in the local community.

Barriers to diagnosis

Overall, nationwide, about a third of those with dementia remain undiagnosed (National Health Service, 2024) and, as noted above, people from some minority ethnic communities may be referred to dementia specialists in lower numbers. In this section, we consider two main sets of barriers to getting a dementia assessment: factors within communities and factors within services. These two types of barriers interact with each other. Both need to be addressed to improve dementia assessment and diagnosis for people from minority ethnic backgrounds.

Community barriers to seeking assessment

As noted in Chapter 3, the early stages of dementia may not be recognized by an individual or their family members due to lack of understanding of the symptoms (Kenning *et al.*, 2017). Initial changes may be dismissed as part of normal ageing or the possibility may be dismissed (Kenning *et al.*, 2017). A Zimbabwean participant in one study (Berwald *et al.*, 2016) declared, 'If I go back to where I was born, you see, dementia, we don't do dementia in our communities' (Berwald *et al.*, 2016, p.7).

For others, the development of cognitive difficulties may be masked by the respect for old age which means older people may not be expected to be very active or independent (Mukadam *et al.*, 2015). An Indian Hindu participant in the study explained that it would not be usual to seek help until very basic activities, such as helping with cooking or taking care of personal hygiene, were affected:

> We have people that...if they have the capacity for the basics...and if that is compromised then that is when we seek care but until then it didn't seem like it was necessary as it wasn't that severe. *(Mukadam et al. 2015, p.6)*

At a point when impairment becomes more obvious, symptoms may not be interpreted as signs of a medical condition but may be attributed to spiritual or other non-medical causes, so families may not seek help from a doctor but from prayer or meditation, or they may ask advice from a religious figure (Regan *et al.*, 2013; Blakemore *et al.*, 2018; Giebel *et al.*, 2019).

It may be an odd or unusual symptom rather than forgetfulness that prompts realization that there is a problem. Mukadam *et al.* (2011) interviewed family carers from 18 families of different ethnicities. Cognitive problems and physical health issues were common triggers for people across all ethnicities to seek help from their doctor but in minority ethnic groups, behavioural problems and safety risks also triggered help-seeking. In the first of the examples below, a person with cognitive problems first realized there was something wrong when she got lost despite being in very familiar surroundings:

> One afternoon, I had just finished a little shopping at Tesco up the road, walking distance; and did not know how to get home. I just could not remember my way home. It was a bit strange. I was just confused. *(Black British individual; Mawaka, 2018, p.79)*

Puzzling or out-of-character behaviours may trigger family members to realize something is wrong:

> So, you say the person is forgetful but when it's getting worse now that she looks in her purse and then she says no, somebody steal something out. You know it's only me and her here and then she says, somebody steals something. *(Black British individual; Mawaka, 2018, p.77)*

> He was...getting quite violent, he was throwing things... I said to the doctor 'Look, you know, my mum can't cope, I can't cope and I'm afraid to leave my mum alone in the house'. *(Asian Bangladeshi individual; Mukadam et al., 2011, p.1073)*

Even when the individual or family members realize something is not right, language, stigma, lack of knowledge about, and distrust of, medical services may still be barriers to seeking assessment.

Older immigrants who do not have wider family to call on may be deterred from seeking medical help because they have difficulty communicating in English. One study found that only 35% of those aged over 65 years in the South Asian community could speak English and only 21% could read and write English (Khan & Tadros, 2014). Equally, first-generation immigrants may lack knowledge of the system and how to negotiate it (Khan & Tadros, 2014; Blakemore *et al.*, 2018).

As noted in Chapter 3, stigma of dementia and of mental illness can place great pressure on individuals and families to hide difficulties. Families may not like the idea of approaching 'outsiders' for help and prefer to cope within the family unless the situation seems risky or is impossible to manage. It has been found that, for people of South Asian backgrounds, the stigma of dementia is a major influence on reluctance to seek help (Hailstone *et al.*, 2017). Social pressure can have more influence than knowledge of dementia or the need to feel in control of the situation. Individuals and families may also be wary due to previous unsatisfactory healthcare encounters and may not trust that they will receive a satisfactory response (Mukadam *et al.*, 2015; Kenning *et al.*, 2017).

Families may equally think there is no point in going to the doctor as there is no cure and the person will be supported in the family anyway, so why go through an assessment. It has been found that White British families value diagnosis in its own right but this is not always the case in Black Caribbean or South Asian families (Mukadam *et al.*, 2011).

Service barriers to assessment

GPs, especially those in less ethnically diverse areas, may not refer minority ethnic people for specialist dementia assessment in the numbers expected, and they may not refer certain ethnicities (Cook *et al.*, 2019). A meta-synthesis of research on barriers and facilitators to people from minority ethnic communities accessing dementia care found a number of service-related barriers (Kenning *et al.*, 2017). Many GPs reinforced the idea of memory loss as a normal part of ageing, which meant carers' concerns were minimized and steps were not taken to assess and diagnose. GPs could be reluctant to pursue dementia diagnosis (Wilson *et al.*, 2020) because they assumed the person would not wish to receive the diagnosis due to stigma (Koch & Iliffe, 2010) or because of their own feelings that a diagnosis was pointless (Moore & Cahill, 2013). In the study by Moore and Cahill, GPs stated that they felt an early diagnosis of dementia was important but were not proactive in referring so that a diagnosis was made. Kenning *et al.* (2017) also concluded that professionals lacked the cultural awareness, specialist knowledge and language abilities needed to manage an accurate assessment and gain a valid diagnosis with people of minority ethnicities.

Ways forward

There have been a number of suggestions about how to overcome the barriers to assessment.

Targeting information about dementia towards specific groups, for example people over 65 years or families that include older people, has produced promising results. Two of the studies summarized in Chapter 3 looked at the impact of a GP sending leaflets about dementia via the post to older people on their lists who were from specific minority ethnic groups. These studies found this encouraged some people to make an GP appointment to address concerns about possible dementia (Mukadam, Cooper & Livingston, 2018; Roche *et al.*, 2018).

To increase trust in health professionals, it may be helpful to offer someone from a minority ethnic group the opportunity to meet a professional from their own community at the GP surgery (Mukadam, Cooper & Livingston, 2018). This is a quote from the family member of a Caribbean man with young onset dementia taken from the Alzheimer's Society report on increasing access to a dementia diagnosis (Arblaster, 2021): 'Having someone from a similar culture and background meant Eugene was much more receptive to care and support' (Arblaster, 2021, p.36).

It may be possible to capitalize on the lack of stigma associated with physical conditions, such as heart disease or diabetes, to provide a route to encouraging help-seeking for cognitive problems. Primary care practitioners supporting people with conditions such as diabetes or asthma could be vigilant to whether the person is developing cognitive problems, and have clear referral pathways for more specialist dementia assessment when this is the case (Alzheimer's Society, 2021).

Kenning *et al.*'s (2017) review includes an excellent schematic diagram that encapsulates what is known about how to address both community and service-related barriers.

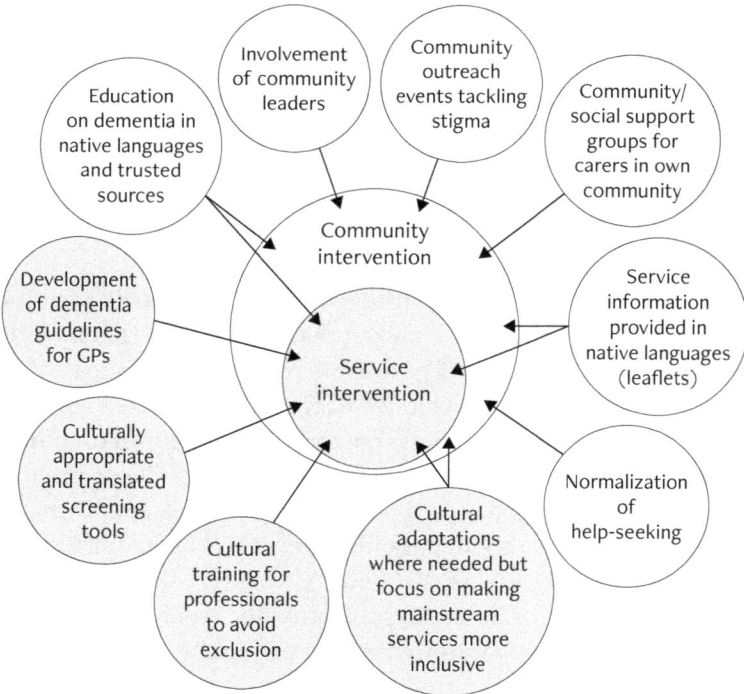

Figure 4.1: *A model for interventions to improve access to dementia assessment and services for people from ethnic minorities in the UK (reproduced from Kenning et al., 2017)*

ACTIVITY 4.2: YOUR PLAN FOR IMPROVING ACCESS TO DEMENTIA ASSESSMENT FOR PEOPLE FROM MINORITY ETHNIC COMMUNITIES

Look at the list of factors outlined by Kenning in the table below and indicate if each is available in your area.

Activity or aspect of service	Is this in place in your area? Yes/No
Involvement with community leaders	
Service information in community languages	
Dementia education from trusted sources in appropriate languages	
Community outreach events to tackle stigma	
Carers support groups in/for ethnic minority communities	
Implementation of strategies that make help-seeking acceptable	
Guidelines for GPs on dementia issues in relation to minority ethnic communities	
Cultural awareness training for professionals	
Cultural adaptations to ensure dementia assessment services are inclusive	
Culturally appropriate screening tools in appropriate languages	

Based on the above, what is one step you could take to improve access to dementia assessment for people from minority ethnic communities?

Dementia assessment

Once the person reaches the point of assessment, there are further considerations to take into account. Diagnosing dementia is not an exact science as there is no definitive single test for its presence. Rather, the diagnosis is based on exclusion of other causes and piecing together evidence from the history, cognitive tests and brain scans. Assessment starts in primary care where a referring GP is expected to gather a good description of cognitive problems, administer a screening test, and carry out blood tests for possible reversible causes before referring on to a specialist assessment service. In the specialist service, members of the multi-disciplinary team carry out a more sophisticated assessment. This usually includes taking a more detailed account of the development of cognitive and functional problems, conducting a more in-depth cognitive assessment, and carrying out a brain scan to see if there is evidence of atrophy (shrinkage) or cardiovascular damage (from mini-strokes). With the exception of the brain scan, the other elements of assessment are strongly influenced by cultural matters, and therefore ethnicity.

Language and interpretation
When meeting a person for assessment, language issues need to be considered first and foremost, as good communication is vital. As noted above, many first-generation immigrants and older people from minority ethnicities do not speak English fluently but also, for those who did acquire English, dementia may lead to its erosion and a return to languages learned earlier in life. Therefore, to communicate effectively the professional either needs to understand and speak the language of the person being assessed or has to rely on an interpreter. The former is clearly preferable as it allows direct communication.

> **POINT FOR PRACTICE: STAFF WHO SPEAK DIFFERENT LANGUAGES**
> Does your employing organization keep a list of its staff who speak different languages? If so, this can be useful to call on to facilitate assessment being conducted by a qualified healthcare professional with language proficiency. If not, could you look into setting one up?

Where interpretation is needed, an older person who does not speak English may feel comfortable depending on a younger family member to interpret. This avoids having to trust a stranger and the older person will be assured that the issues discussed will remain in the family. However, there are some disadvantages. This could invade the person's privacy and possibly disturb family relationships. In addition, the relative is not likely to be knowledgeable about dementia assessment, so they may not have the expertise to interpret questions meaningfully from English to the language of the person being assessed; also, due to shame or stigma, the family member may not translate fully the responses of the person being assessed. A professional interpreter brings some advantages. They are more able to remain emotionally neutral compared with a relative; most interpreters have a specialist qualification in health interpreting or have developed specialist vocabulary, and they follow professional guidelines about how to be an effective intermediary. The summary of an extensive Alzheimer's Europe report on providing timely assessment and diagnosis across ethnicities concludes that clinicians should 'Not ask relatives and friends to act as interpreters, except for emergencies or exceptionally, but to consult them during the assessment process if required and subject to the agreement of the person being assessed' (Gove et al., 2021, p.1826).

Cultural aspects of interviewing and history-taking

Values and norms about interaction and conversation differ across cultures, concerning who should be present, who should speak, greetings and what is acceptable to talk about. In majority British culture, it is widely accepted that:

- to stand and offer a handshake is a respectful greeting
- an older person should first be addressed as Miss, Mrs or Mr and their surname before a first name is used
- the person being assessed should speak for themselves
- direct questions about personal matters are expected when talking with a doctor, whether that person is of the same gender or not.

These conventions often differ for people from different ethnicities.

> **POINT FOR PRACTICE: GREETINGS**
> For one or two of the main minority ethnicities in your local population:
>
> - Find out how it is expected you should greet people on first meeting.
> - If you do not know the greeting in the appropriate language already, then learn it.
> - Find out the convention about how to address older people.

To take a good history and gain an accurate description of current cognitive and functional difficulties, there is a need for open communication. However, not only may stigma and shame lead the person and family members to minimize difficulties but also speaking about personal matters to someone outside the family may not be considered wise or safe. In addition, some immigrants may have had traumatic life experiences in conflict zones or circumstances of deprivation or poverty before coming to the UK and many will have experienced overt or more subtle racism during their years in the UK. This may mean some find it difficult to revisit the past and some may be reluctant to reveal information that could put them in a vulnerable position. If there are gaps in the information obtained, clinical experience suggests it is important to keep an open mind about the potential reasons rather than assume these gaps arise due to memory difficulties.

Issues of privacy and distrust of strangers make it vital to take time to build trusting relationships. It may be tempting to manage by talking primarily to a family member rather than directly to the person concerned. An experienced professional interviewed for the ADAPT study spoke of the emphasis she places on this. She says she finds it more valuable to gain a history than to have a cognitive assessment: 'It's so much more, I guess, important and valid to listen to the collective history that been given by the caregiver and I guess all the other background information that's being given at the assessment.'

However, it remains important to hear directly the voice of the person themselves as their experience and perspective may differ from that of family members.

Over time, many healthcare professionals become familiar with common examples of how cognitive impairment is noticed, for example forgetting appointments, getting lost in the local shopping centre or burning pans on the stove. When working with particular ethnicities, health and care staff find they build familiarity with culturally specific examples, such as forgetting a sequence of prayers, or adding salt several times when preparing food.

> **POINT FOR PRACTICE: EARLY SIGNS IN ETHNIC MINORITY GROUPS**
> Could you discuss in your team your various experiences of how early signs of cognitive impairment have impacted on everyday activities in minority ethnic groups in your local area? This may help to sensitize you to areas to enquire about or listen out for when taking a history.

Cognitive screening and assessment

The need for valid cognitive screening and assessment tools is one of the most visited issues concerning dementia and ethnicity. The problems of using tests devised and normed with White British (or indeed American) populations are well rehearsed. A number of barriers to validity are shown in the table below.

Table 4.1: Barriers to the validity of cognitive assessments for minority ethnic populations

Factors related to the individual being assessed
May not understand or speak fluent English.
May have had little formal education, therefore may not be literate and not have assumed knowledge.
May not use paper and pencil in day-to-day life, so are disadvantaged by paper and pencil items in tests.

cont.

Different life experiences lead to different culturally based knowledge. What is assumed to be universal may not apply and, conversely, culturally based strengths may not be tapped in 'western' tests.

Ethnicity is not the only influence on appropriateness of cognitive screening tests. The influence of ethnicity intersects with other factors such as sensory functioning and physical health.

Factors related to the nature of the test items

Items may be obviously culturally biased, for example asking the person to identify fragmented letters of the British alphabet.

Items may be more subtly culturally biased, such as asking a person to recall 'apple–table–penny' or judging object naming by asking the person to identify line drawings of animals and objects common in British culture and books, such as a camel or a ship's anchor.

Items may be very subtly culturally biased – asking the person to copy shapes (an activity that is more familiar in western than African or Asian cultures) or to draw a clock face.

Factors related to normative performance

Cut-off scores for presence of impairment are likely to be based on predominantly White indigenous samples.

Thorough translation of languages does not equate to cultural translation of items.

It is vital to consider these limitations when selecting cognitive screening instruments and interpreting their scores. Tests that are not culturally validated are poorer at discriminating between minority ethnic people with and without cognitive impairment and result in both false negatives and false positives (i.e., some people without dementia score as if they have impairment and some who do have dementia are not identified).

Cognitive screening in primary care

Within primary care, NICE guidance recommends that practitioners use one of six brief cognitive screening instruments (NICE, 2018). Each yields a single score that can be judged against cut-off points. Most are reliant on use of English and influenced by UK education and familiarity with British (or US) culture; for example, the Six Item Cognitive Impairment Test (6-CIT) requires the person to say the months of the year backwards, while the Mini-Cog includes clock drawing. The Memory Impairment Screen (Buschke et al., 1999; Kuslansky et al., 2002), a four-minute test of learning and memory, has been described as the most appropriate for people from minority ethnicities and is recommended by the Alzheimer's Society (2021). It is brief, does not require writing and is less influenced by education and language than most other brief cognitive screening tests (Cordell et al., 2013). However, the words to be learned and recalled are heavily culturally loaded (the four in the main version are: checkers, saucer, telegram, Red Cross) so this cannot be recommended as culture-free; also, the person being assessed is expected to be able to read the four words.

> **POINT FOR PRACTICE: LIMITATIONS OF BRIEF COGNITIVE SCREENING TESTS**
>
> In light of the above, brief cognitive screening tests and their results should be considered with extreme caution if the individual does not have English as a first language, was not educated beyond primary school or did not grow up in the UK.

Cognitive assessment in dementia assessment services

Within dementia assessment services, multi-domain cognitive tests, such as the Addenbrooke's Cognitive Examination (ACE) (Hodges & Larner, 2017) and the Montreal Cognitive Assessment (MoCA) (Nasreddine et al., 2005), are usually used to obtain a fuller picture of cognitive functioning. These provide scores for different domains such as attention, memory, word fluency, language abilities and visuo-spatial functioning. The original English language versions of both the ACE and the MoCA are culturally rooted. A clinical psychologist interviewed as part of the ADAPT study summarized her view: 'They're very, very English focused and a lot of the language that they use and the words they ask you to remember and the pictures...'

However, considerable attempts have been made to translate and culturally adapt both tests. A systematic review of ACE adaptations located 32, including 17 for the ACE-III (the most up-to-date version), across a range of cultures and languages including Arabic, South Asian, South-East Asian and European (Waheed *et al.*, 2020). An equivalent review of the MoCA located 86 adaptations (Cova *et al.*, 2022). To adapt a cognitive test thoroughly, so it yields reliable, valid results for a particular population, is a complex, painstaking process (Waheed *et al.*, 2020; Khan, Mirza & Waheed, 2022). An article about the development of an Urdu version of the ACE-III for UK use gives in-depth insights into this process; for example, the British South Asian sample preferred some words to be transliterated from English to Urdu script rather than translated (e.g., participants preferred 'ball' to be spelt out in Urdu script, not translated into the Urdu word for ball) (Mirza, Panagioti & Waheed, 2018).

An alternative to translating and adapting tests is to design them as 'culture fair' by trying to avoid cultural influences. The Rowland Universal Dementia Assessment Scale (RUDAS) (Rowland *et al.*, 2006) is currently the most prominent of these. It was developed in Australia and has been validated there and across a range of immigrant populations in a number of European countries (Nielsen & Jørgensen, 2020) but not in a UK sample, as far as we know. Its items were selected to be valid across cultures. Its accuracy is not affected by language or gender but has been found to be affected by education, so it is important to use education-adjusted cut-off points (Nielsen & Jørgensen, 2020).

Given the challenges to reliability and validity of cognitive tests when used with minority ethnic populations in the UK, it would be easy to back away from using them at all. However, they do give the clinician an idea about how each individual responds in a situation where they need to find answers – something that is very hard to pick up accurately from an interview with the person or their family. The scores need to be treated sceptically but can be valuable for the qualitative information they provide and can give a baseline against which to compare later assessments to check for changes over time.

> **POINT FOR PRACTICE: DEMENTIA ASSESSMENT TESTS FOR THE SOUTH ASIAN COMMUNITIES**
> The recent ADAPT study recommended the ACE, MoCA or RUDAS as the three preferred options for use in dementia assessment with South Asian people in the UK. See https://raceequalityfoundation.org.uk/adapt for details and resources.

Functional assessment

A further component of dementia assessment is to establish, at first hand, the person's ability to carry out activities of daily living. This is often addressed by occupational therapists observing the person making a snack or a drink. This is an activity that sounds simple but actually involves a sequence of steps that draw on different cognitive functions. However, as with cognitive assessments, it is vital to think about how an activity is influenced by culture before using it in assessment. An occupational therapist interviewed as part of the ADAPT study commented on how commonly she had seen making beans on toast used within the Assessment of Motor and Process Skills (AMPS) tool (Fischer, 2001): 'I don't remember seeing any, for want of a better word, snack-based tasks that were not making beans on toast, which are obviously very much a British snack-based food.'

> **POINT FOR PRACTICE: USING THE ASSESSMENT OF MOTOR AND PROCESS SKILLS**
> The instructions for the AMPS state that tasks to be assessed should be agreed between the assessor and the person and should be things they used to do that are both relevant and meaningful to them. Making sure you discuss this with individuals from minority ethnicities who are having an assessment will help to ensure that your assessment is valid.

Speaking with family members

Due to the limitations of standardized cognitive assessments in British minority ethnic groups, gaining a clear account of the situation from knowledgeable family members is even more important than in the White British population. A professional interviewed as part of the ADAPT study stressed the place of this within assessment:

> The clinical history and the understanding of the development of the difficulties, the onset, the trajectory, the main issues at hand, that feels to me more valuable information for diagnostic accuracy than a cognitive score.

In a White British nuclear family, there is usually one individual, a spouse, partner or adult-child, who is the key supporter. In some minority ethnic communities, the person is more likely to have an extended family structure, which makes the situation more complex; so the practitioner should pay attention to the role of the spokesperson. Sometimes, a male family member is seen as the appropriate spokesperson to liaise with professionals, so it could be, for example, that a son attends the appointment but that hands-on care and support are being provided by a daughter and/or daughter-in-law. By contrast, some older people from minority ethnicities may be living alone and have no informant to give detailed information. This would be the case, for example, for those who immigrated alone and have remained isolated in the UK or for those who are separated or divorced and do not have close contact with any adult children.

The ADAPT study, which consulted widely with people of South Asian ethnicity as well as professionals about the South Asian care pathway in the UK, proposed that the Alzheimer's Questionnaire (Malek-Ahmadi *et al.*, 2012) could be used as a proxy cognitive assessment in the South Asian community. This 21-item questionnaire was developed in the US to provide a systematic overview of cognitive functioning from an informant's point of view and has been validated in India but not, to date, in the UK. The score indicates presence of dementia, mild cognitive impairment or normal cognitive functioning.

> **POINT FOR PRACTICE: TAKING A HISTORY**
> If you are taking a history from family members, find out how much the family member knows first-hand about the situation. Where more information is needed, see if you can speak with the direct carers or ask to have a family meeting, possibly by a home visit.

Conclusion

In the first part of this chapter, we summarized evidence about assessment and diagnosis of dementia for people from minority ethnicities. The research shows that this is complex. We cannot generalize across or even within minority ethnic groups; ethnicity does not stand alone but 'intersects' with other characteristics, and the position is constantly changing given our dynamic society.

In the second part, we described community barriers to people coming forward for assessment: lack of awareness and knowledge, viewing changes as due to normal ageing or spiritual causes, stigma, and distrust of services. We also reflected on service-related barriers in primary care, including GPs' reluctance to refer for specialist assessment, for fear of causing offence due to stigma. You should now be more aware of ways to overcome these barriers, including through targeted awareness campaigns, information leaflets for older people from their GPs or trusted community members, and offering clinics for people with language abilities and shared cultural backgrounds.

In the third part, we covered considerations across the assessment process, including issues around language and interpretation; cultural aspects around interviewing and history-taking; cognitive screening; and cognitive and functional assessment. We hope you now feel you know more about how to communicate effectively with people from minority ethnicities during assessment and how to assess in a culturally appropriate way so that you can have confidence in your assessment results and your diagnosis.

In the next chapter, we move on to the post-diagnostic period and look at living with dementia in the community.

Chapter 5

Living with Dementia in the Community

I do think, you shouldn't be embarrassed to ask for help, you should try and get whatever help is out there and you should absolutely explore all your options and utilise what is there to help you.

(SOUTH ASIAN DAUGHTER-IN-LAW, INTERVIEWED FOR THE CAREGIVING HOPE STUDY)

Introduction

It is a common misconception that the majority of people living with dementia reside in care homes. In reality, 80% of people living with dementia continue to live in the community, often with family support. Research suggests that by 2040, almost 38% of people with dementia living within the community will be solely relying on support from family members and friends (Wittenberg *et al.*, 2019). In this chapter, we consider caregiving and family dynamics in minority communities and reflect on common cultural stereotypes such as 'they look after their own'. We also establish the barriers families experience in accessing health and social care services and how these can be overcome. We consider interventions and therapeutic approaches to enable families to live as well as possible with dementia, and finally we explore the importance of cultural competence for health and social care practitioners.

Caregiving and family dynamics

Alzheimer's Research UK published a report in 2015, outlining the impact of dementia on family carers. Alzheimer's Research UK predicts that there are approximately 700,000 relatives who are providing unpaid care and support to family members living with dementia. The report goes on to outline the negative impact this 'caregiving role' can have on the relatives' physical and psychological health, the significant financial burden, with many carers needing to give up employment, and the social isolation experienced by carers. While the negative impact of caregiving on relatives has been well documented in research, there is evidence to suggest that caregiving can also be a positive experience for family members. For example, a review of 81 studies, including 3347 carers, concluded that family carers can experience a strengthening of family relationships and also gain confidence in personal accomplishments such as learning new skills as a result of caregiving (Lindeza et al., 2020).

It is difficult to establish the number of relatives providing care to a person living with dementia from minority ethnic backgrounds due to a number of reasons. The term 'carer' is often not used within minority ethnic families, as 'caregiving' is often seen as normal family responsibility. Furthermore, dementia remains stigmatized within these communities, and family members do not disclose that they are caregiving for a relative with dementia. This multiple jeopardy experienced by minority ethnic families means they often experience a worse quality of life than White British carers.

Who is the carer?

It is often assumed that there is a primary carer for a person living with dementia at home. This is often not the case for minority ethnic families, where a number of people may be involved with the care, with each member taking responsibility for specific tasks. In South Asian households, it may be the eldest male who is the decision maker and often labelled as the 'primary carer' but in reality, the day-to-day care may be provided by the daughters and daughters-in-law. In our Caregiving HOPE study, which included over 700 White British and South Asian carers, we found that South Asian carers were more likely to be:

- adult children
- female
- younger
- caring for other dependents (e.g., young children)
- caring for more hours.

> **POINT FOR PRACTICE: IDENTIFYING THE CARERS**
> Given differences in family structures and norms for some minority ethnic families, it is important to ask about who provides support for the person with dementia, and to find out if different aspects of support are offered by different family members. Using this information, everyone who is involved can be included in care planning.

Cultural and religious influences on family care

It is worth noting that religion and cultural values may also influence the type of care family members can provide (Hossain & Khan, 2020). For example, in a Muslim household, adult children can only provide personal care to the same-gender parent. In the Caregiving HOPE study, we spoke to a son who had to seek special dispensation from a mufti (a religious leader) in order to support his mother's personal care:

> He (the mufti) said they could hear mum, because they're next door neighbours. She needs 24/7 care, so yes you are permitted to do that. So, the fact that he has given the blessings to do it, I'm still conscious of what the community will think.

Perhaps due to the complex family dynamics of minority ethnic communities, there is a prevalent misconception that minority ethnic families 'look after their own', and perhaps don't require external support and services. It is true that our cultural values influence whether we become 'carers' and shape the caregiving experience, from how we perceive the role (whether it is considered burdensome or a role with positive aspects), how we cope with the role and the impact on quality of life. There are three key constructs to consider when exploring how ethnicity may impact on the caregiving role and the person with dementia.

These are:

- *Traditional care ideology:* Caregiving is seen as a natural part of the relationship and virtuous. The traditional ideology implies that family members give priority to those who need support, even if this is at some cost to the individual well-being of those providing care and support. A South Asian carer in the Caregiving HOPE study spoke about traditional care ideology within Islam: 'There is a duty as a Muslim and as a son, to look after the parents, no matter what.'

- *Familism:* Similar to traditional care ideology, familism is a construct that captures the value placed on solidarity and loyalty among family members. Those with high familism feel closely connected and are strongly attached to their family, both nuclear and extended. Where there is a high degree of familism, families are described as holding strong feelings of loyalty, providing mutual support and having solidarity with each other. A South Asian carer in the Caregiving HOPE study discussed familism:

My own parents, would, would be absolutely horrified if that had happened [if a parent had been moved to a care home]. My dad used to care for my grandfather. My grandfather didn't live with us. All the relatives had a house on the same road, so there'd be like, everyone would be popping in and out, kind of thing...but I, my mindset and my attitude and all of that, is, you know, they're your parents at the end of the day, so you care for them, full stop.

- *Xiao (translated as filial piety):* A different but overlapping construct that captures power dynamics, obligations and reciprocity within parent–child relationships is that of xiao or filial piety. This reflects the Confucian ethics that shape Chinese-related cultures and embodies the view that a stable society is sustained through the younger generation supporting and succeeding the older generation. It has been suggested that the construct has two dimensions: authoritarian filial piety, which involves respect and obedience from a child to a parent, who carries authority, and reciprocal filial piety, which involves the idea that children repay their parents for care given to them in childhood by caring for them in turn as they grow older. In this quote from a PhD study by Oladayo Bifarin, a young Chinese graduate living in the UK gives her view, demonstrating the reciprocal dimension of xiao:

It's not something about confidence, is something about duty, about responsibility, I think if they provide their love to us, I just have to pay back, no matter what I think. It's a duty for me, a real responsible person, a social person, not to try to avoid responsibilities. I just imagine, if I have some serious disease, would my parents just say I will not take care of this kid? No, they wouldn't. So, I based on this assumption, I will provide my xiao to them, in any circumstances. (Bifarin, 2022)

There is significant research to suggest that minority ethnic carers have higher levels of familism and filial piety compared to carers from western cultures. In America, considerable research has found that African-American, Hispanic and South Korean carers have higher levels of familism than White American carers (Youn et al., 1999; Kim, Knight & Longmire, 2007; Sayegh & Knight, 2013; Cahill et al., 2021). In the UK, our research has also found that South Asian carers have higher levels of familism than White British carers (Parveen, Morrison & Robinson, 2013). So why is 'they look after their own' a myth? Research suggests that although family members may feel culturally obligated to provide care, this may not always be possible in practical terms. Family structures of South Asian families have changed considerably over the last 20 years, and the nuclear family has become the norm rather than the traditional extended family. Due to changing economic pressures and immigration policies, family members have become separated over larger geographical regions; for example, sons and daughters may now have to move away from their parents in order to find suitable employment. They may still feel culturally obligated to provide care, but it is no longer practically possible.

Motivations, willingness and preparedness to care

Cultural values are only one factor that influences whether a family member adopts the caregiver role. Two types of motivations have been proposed to influence whether a family member adopts the care role: extrinsic and intrinsic motivations (Lyonette & Yardley, 2003).

- *Extrinsic motivations:* feeling as if you have no choice, feeling obligated or caregiving out of guilt.
- *Intrinsic motivations:* caregiving because you have a caring nature, because you love the person or because you are an altruistic person.

Lyonette and Yardley's work with family carers of older people has found that those who are intrinsically motivated to care experience less burden and have a more positive relationship with the older person. Those who are extrinsically motivated experience more burden in their role and poorer health for the carer and the older person. Our work with South Asian and White British carers of relatives living with dementia suggests that while a carer's cultural values have influence on their experience of caregiving, other factors also come into play. A carer may feel culturally obligated to provide care but may also feel unwilling to provide it. Another carer may feel very willing to provide care to a family member but unprepared for the various aspects of the caregiving role.

ACTIVITY 5.1: MOTIVATIONS FOR CARE

Read the case studies below and consider what has motivated the carer to provide support to a relative living with dementia, and how willing and prepared they are.

After you have thought about your suggestions, have a look at our ideas at the end of this chapter.

Kiran is 38 years of age and the eldest daughter in the family. She has been providing care for her mother for the last three years. Kiran has two younger brothers but they live abroad so Kiran felt there was no other option but for her to be the main carer. She was happy for her mum to move in with her and to do the everyday tasks such as cooking and cleaning but she struggles with the emotional care and sometimes finds it a burden having to constantly reassure her mum. She is often anxious about how the dementia will progress and what her role will involve. She doesn't currently need to provide personal care but realizes she may need to in the future and is unsure if she is ready.

Jamal is 25 years of age and the only son in his family. His father has just been diagnosed with young onset dementia. Jamal is very happy to provide care for his dad; he believes it his duty to care for his parents and he wants to pay his dad back for everything he has done for him. He is very willing to provide emotional and practical support. He is unsure what type of support his dad will need, and he hasn't done any research. He believes that supporting his dad will be straightforward and as long as he is organized, he will manage just fine.

Anne is 67 years of age and has been providing care for her mum for two years now. Initially, Anne was happy to become her mum's main carer, as Anne had just retired from nursing and her younger sister was still working. She also felt she had more of a caring personality and it was in her nature to care for others. However, her mum's needs have become complex quite quickly and she is less sure about being the main carer. She had expected the changes and with her nursing background, she had felt ready to manage them. Anne finds herself sometimes feeling a little resentful, as soon she will need to move in with her mum and she is not keen on the idea. She had planned to travel during her retirement and experience new things but now feels robbed of her retirement.

It is important to remember that motivations, willingness and preparedness to care change over time and this will have an impact on the family. Consider the following case. We met Subitha in 2017

as part of the Caregiving HOPE study. Her mum had recently been diagnosed with early onset Alzheimer's disease. Subitha and her four siblings had decided they would care for and support their mother at home. We asked her if they would consider a care home for their mum as a future care option. Her response:

> No! Absolutely not. My mum would never just throw me in a care home, my mum would never just wash her hands of us. No way, she's my own flesh and blood. She gave me life, my brothers and sisters have had this discussion, we sat and talked about her changing needs, and one of the topics that did come up was about having extra carers in or possibly looking at a care home. Everybody decided hell no. She will never ever go into a care home.

We met with Subitha again 12 months later and asked her the same question. Her response:

> Things are difficult now. She gets agitated and I just can't calm her down. My siblings aren't always around and I can't cope by myself. In fact, just before you came I was actually googling how to look for a care home...yeah, things are that bad now.

> **POINT FOR REFLECTION: CHANGES IN WILLINGNESS AND PREPAREDNESS OVER TIME**
> How willing and prepared was Subitha in 2017? Had these feelings changed by 2018?

In the Caregiving HOPE study, of 700 White British and South Asian carers, we found that cultural obligation and willingness to care were associated with carer outcomes such as burden, anxiety and depression. However, the best predictor of carers' outcomes was how prepared carers felt; for example, the more prepared carers thought they were for the caregiving role in 2017, the less likely they were to experience burden and be anxious and depressed in 2018. This suggests that by preparing family members for the caregiver role, we can support them to have a more positive and less burdensome experience. In 2013, the Carers Trust published a report, *A Road Less Rocky*, outlining ten 'stress trigger points' for carers of people living with dementia (Newbronner *et al.*, 2013) (see Activity 5.2).

ACTIVITY 5.2: PREPARING FOR TRANSITION POINTS

Below are the ten stress trigger points for dementia carers identified by the Carers Trust (Newbronner *et al.*, 2013).

1. When dementia is diagnosed
2. When the carer takes on an active role
3. When the capacity of the person with dementia declines
4. When the carer needs a break
5. When the person with dementia loses their mobility
6. When the person with dementia has other health problems
7. When the carer has to cope with behavioural problems
8. When the carer's own circumstances change
9. When the person with dementia becomes incontinent
10. When decisions about residential and end-of-life care have to be made

How can we support and prepare carers for each of these transition points in dementia care?

How can current approaches be made more culturally sensitive for diverse populations?

Living well with dementia

A person-centred holistic approach to dementia care means that people living with dementia and their families are supported not only by health services but also by social care and third-sector community organizations. There is an increasing focus on enabling families to 'live well' with dementia, with living well often being equated with a good quality of life. Quinn *et al.* (2022) suggest six key considerations that influence a person's capability to live well with dementia:

1. Psychological characteristics (outlook on life)
2. Physical health and level of physical fitness
3. Level of social engagement
4. Independence in daily activities
5. Quality of relationships and feelings of loneliness
6. Perceived social standing and perceived role in society

A person's ability to live well with dementia will very much depend on the individual and their circumstances. When considering people living with dementia from minority ethnic backgrounds, the factors described above may impede people from living well with dementia. For example, as discussed in Chapter 2, people from minority ethnic communities may have poor physical health and live with multiple co-morbidities such as diabetes and hypertension. Stigma (see Chapter 3) may lead to a negative social standing and a diminished role in society. One study compared 20 minority ethnic people affected by dementia in the UK with 60 White British people affected by dementia and found that those from minority ethnicities experienced lower relationship quality, higher levels of loneliness and stress and a poorer quality of life (Victor *et al.*, 2024).

A large UK study asked 1339 people living with dementia, 'What does living well (with dementia) mean to you?' (Quinn *et al.*, 2022). Activity 5.3 focuses on their findings.

ACTIVITY 5.3: LIVING WELL WITH DEMENTIA

These were the top responses to the question 'What does living well (with dementia) mean to you? (Quinn *et al.*, 2022).

- Being engaged and having an active lifestyle
- Positive relationships with others
- Good living situation/environment
- Having security
- Getting on with life
- Being able to get out and about
- A positive outlook on life
- Being able to cope

- Having independence
- Having a purpose

Reflect: Can you pick three aspects from this list that would be especially important to you, if you were to have a diagnosis of dementia?

In 2024, we conducted workshops with 40 South Asian and 40 African or Caribbean people affected by dementia and asked the following two questions: 'Do you think it's possible to live well with dementia?' and 'What would enable people in your community to live well with dementia?' All those from South Asian backgrounds believed that it was possible to live well with dementia, if the family had the 'right support' from services. Those from African and Caribbean backgrounds thought that while it may be possible to live well with dementia, their communities were 'not ready for these conversations'. They believed that significant dementia awareness and basic dementia education were needed within their communities before they could begin to have conversations about how to live well with dementia. In response to the second question, 'What would enable people in your community to live well with dementia?', participants believed that families would need information and support with the following topics:

- Healthy diet/nutrition
- How to keep physically active
- How to keep the brain healthy and active
- Keeping socially engaged
- Managing complex needs when the person has advanced dementia
- Communicating effectively with the person living with dementia
- Legal and financial advice
- Managing relationships with extended family members and friends

All participants believed that post-diagnostic support and information were key to enable families to live well with dementia. While those from a South Asian background wanted post-diagnostic support and information to be provided by GP surgeries and community groups, those from African and Caribbean backgrounds preferred the information to be provided by their church leaders.

As part of the ADAPT project, we reviewed which evidence-based post-diagnostic support and interventions had been culturally adapted and made available for South Asian families. We found very few examples of culturally adapted interventions and many had not been implemented beyond a small locality. These examples can be found within the ADAPT toolkit (just scan the QR code with your phone)[1].

Promising examples included information programmes for carers and cognitive stimulation therapy for people living with dementia. Cognitive stimulation therapy is currently undergoing cultural adaptation for different ethnic communities as part of a large programme of work (Spector *et al.*, 2019; Morrish *et al.*, 2022). If successful, it is hoped that this intervention will be made available for more people from diverse minority ethnic groups. There is evidence to suggest that by culturally adapting interventions, we can enhance their effectiveness (Akarsu *et al.*, 2019).

Access to support

While there is a growing acknowledgement that post-diagnostic support needs to be culturally adapted to meet the needs of families affected by dementia, current research suggests that minority ethnic communities continue to experience barriers in accessing available treatment and support to enable them to live well with dementia. Barriers to post-diagnostic support services can be categorized at three levels:

1. *Individual-level barriers:* A person may be unaware of the specialist dementia services that exist in their area, and they mistrust health and social care professionals.
2. *Community-level barriers:* There is a perceived stigma for

---

[1] https://raceequalityfoundation.org.uk/adapt/the-toolkit/psychosocial-interventions-for-people-living-with-dementia-and-their-families-from-south-asian-communities

the person living with dementia and/or their family members in using post-diagnostic dementia support services.
3. *Service-level barriers:* Services not providing culturally sensitive care, lack of translators or racism.

In 2020, we reviewed all the research focusing on the barriers and facilitators for minority ethnic communities when attempting to access specialist dementia services. Based on the most common barriers reported, we produced the following recommendations:

1. Rather that creating new services, existing services should be culturally adapted to meet the needs of a diverse community.
2. Existing evidence-based therapies such as cognitive stimulation therapy should be culturally adapted and made available on a wider scale.
3. Services should be co-designed with the community.
4. Health and social care professionals should take an active role in promoting and raising awareness of available dementia services.
5. Bilingual dementia workers are vital in building trusting relationships with the community.
6. Access to interpreters should be an underpinning service principle.
7. Dementia services are more effective when there is partnership working between health, social and community-based care.
8. Training and workforce development is required as a number of health and social care professionals report a lack of confidence and knowledge to work with those with language or cultural differences.

Carers UK (2023) provided further general (not dementia-specific) guidance on supporting family carers from a minority ethnic background. The guidance included the following points:

- *When providing information and advice:* Translate information, use interpreters where possible, include diverse

language and imagery, use the appropriate terminology, avoid stereotypes, and make use of bilingual staff to disseminate information.
- *When providing culturally sensitive services:* Take the time to understand different cultures and values, work in partnership with organizations that have expertise in working with the community of interest, mark special events such as Black History Month, and provide safe spaces for staff and carers to discuss race and culture.
- *To improve health and well-being of carers:* Take a holistic approach, form specific networks and groups focusing on a particular minority community, and address issues such as psychological health and social isolation.
- *Create a diverse and inclusive workforce:* Provide training on culturally competent care.
- *Involve minority ethnic carers in policy and practice:* co-design polices and services.

> **POINT FOR PRACTICE: INCLUSIVE COMMUNITY SERVICES**
> Considering the recommendations above, what changes can you introduce to your service to ensure that it is inclusive and meets the needs of minority ethnic communities?

Cultural competence for practitioners

As we have outlined above, while minority ethnic families do believe that it is possible to live well with dementia in the community, this requires culturally competent support from health and social care practitioners. A key barrier for minority ethnic families affected by dementia in accessing the community services they require is the lack of culturally sensitive support and a mistrust of health and social care professionals. Cultural competency is key for health and social care professionals in order to provide care that is tailored to the family's values and needs.

Cultural competency also promotes person-centred approaches that promote trust and collaboration between services providers and families.

Recently there has been a rise in cultural competency training for health and social care professionals but the quality and impact of this training remains uncertain. A review of literature on cultural competency training (Brottman *et al.*, 2020) proposed that all health and social care providers should be educated on:

- health inequalities and disparities
- the needs of diverse populations
- unconscious bias
- advocacy.

In 2016, the Department of Health, in collaboration with Health Education England, published a Dementia Core Skills Education and Training Framework, revised in 2018 to become the Dementia Training Standards Framework (Skills for Health, 2018). The framework stipulates that all health and social care professionals who have direct contact with people living with dementia must complete at least tier 2 of training. This includes a module on 'Equality, Diversity and Inclusion in Dementia Care', commissioned from us at the University of Bradford, which covers the main elements of cultural competency training.

Brottman and colleagues' review investigated the most effective educational strategies for cultural competency training across 89 studies (Brottman *et al.*, 2020). They identified 11 commonly used strategies: immersive experiences, simulation, discussion groups (small and large), lectures, reflection, e-learning, case-based learning, reading, writing papers, attending presentations and watching videos. The review did not provide conclusive evidence about the most effective learning strategy but did report that cultural competency training was found to benefit the health and social care workforce and the families they supported. Table 5.1 shows ten tips you can use to help you develop your own cultural competency.

Table 5.1: Ten top tips for your cultural competency learning journey

1	Learn about your own historical roots, beliefs and values. Reflect on how these values influence how you and your family function as a group.
2	Interact with diverse groups and learn about different cultures. Value diversity.
3	Attend diversity-focused events and conferences.
4	Be adaptable – people perceive the world differently, so be open to this.
5	Ask lots of questions and actively listen to diverse communities.
6	Eliminate communication bias. Think about the language you use and the different modes you use to communicate. Is your language or mode of communication excluding any particular groups?
7	Promote culturally sensitive communication skills in your team and organization.
8	Understand cultural cues, such as not shaking a Muslim woman's hand unless they offer their hand.
9	Be aware of traditional holidays.
10	Practise empathic attunement (meet people in their world).

Conclusion

The majority of people living with dementia continue to live within the community with support from family members and friends. However, those who feel culturally obligated to provide care may not always be willing to provide care and support or may feel unprepared for the carer role. In order to live as well as possible with dementia within the community, minority ethnic families require culturally adapted post-diagnostic support services and evidence-based therapies such as cognitive stimulation therapy. They face a number of barriers when trying to access support, which could be mitigated by a culturally competent dementia care workforce. While many minority ethnic families may feel more culturally obligated to provide care and support at home than the majority, they may not always be able to fulfil these obligations. In the next chapter, we move on to consider ethnic minority issues in relation to use of care homes.

> **REFLECTIONS ON ACTIVITY 5.1**
> These three carers differ in their motivations, willingness and how prepared they are.
>
> Kiran is extrinsically motivated, willing but unprepared. Her motivation is external as she had no choice about becoming her mum's carer. Despite this, she was willing to take this on, saying she was happy for her mum to move in. However, she struggles with emotional care and does not feel she is ready to provide personal care, so is not prepared.
>
> Jamal is both extrinsically and intrinsically motivated, and is willing but very unprepared. His main motivation is feeling it is his duty (external) but he also wants to repay his dad (internal). He expresses willingness to care for his dad but he clearly has not accessed any information about what is involved.
>
> Anne is intrinsically motivated and prepared but has become less willing over time. Her initial motivation came from her sense of herself as caring and her altruism as she was in a better position to care than her sister. She is prepared, in that she has knowledge and experience from her nursing career. However, she has shifted from initial willingness to a position of some resentment.

Chapter 6

Using Care Homes

> Wherever we went there wasn't a single person that was Pakistani, Asian, Muslim, whatever. So that's an issue because they didn't really understand her needs, cultural, dietary, religious and so on. We found one place, and within one day we got a call from the place saying, 'We can't cope with your mum's needs, can you take her? We can't cope with her needs, she's disturbing the other residents, can you take her home?'
>
> (FAMILY CARER; CAREGIVING HOPE STUDY)

Introduction

This chapter considers residential care homes and what is important for culturally appropriate care in these settings. The chapter is divided into two main sections.

In the first section, 'Deciding whether to use a care home', we consider the reasons why people from minority ethnic backgrounds use care homes, look at whether attitudes to residential care are changing and give examples of how families cope with the stigma that can arise if a person with dementia moves into care.

In the second section, 'Living in a care home', we present statistics on how many people from minority ethnic communities live in care homes and consider important issues in providing culturally appropriate care for people of diverse ethnicities, including communication, food, social connections and activities, faith and racism.

By the end of this chapter, you should have a good understanding of why people from minority ethnic populations may decide to use care homes, and have gained some ideas about how to provide care that caters for their cultural needs.

Deciding whether to use a care home

There are two types of care homes in the UK: residential care homes focus on personal care, whereas nursing homes provide personal care and 24-hour, on-site nursing care. Many people with dementia who move to a care home have advanced dementia that is affecting cognitive and verbal communication abilities and ability to self-care. The person may have mobility problems, swallowing difficulties or incontinence. Due to these significant care needs, those with advanced dementia are likely to move into a nursing home. In this chapter, we refer to care homes as a generic term that encompasses residential and nursing homes, unless there is reason to make the distinction.

Despite the cultural value placed on providing care at home and people's willingness to do so, it is not always possible or desirable to continue to care at home. In this section, we look at what may prompt people from minority ethnic backgrounds to use care homes. First, we describe examples where use of a care home is seen as acceptable because there are issues around abuse. We then consider the influences of societal and generational changes on attitudes to care. Finally, we look at how families who use care homes manage the stigma linked with acting in a way that is not seen as consistent with community values.

Abusive situations

People we have spoken with from a range of minority ethnic communities suggest that an abusive situation at home would justify using a care home. The quote below is from an interview with a man of Indian origin. He was fully committed to caring for his father at home but he expressed the view that in a situation where there is abuse, it would be appropriate for the person to move to a care home. He related this to an example of an older person who was neglected by family:

> When you send families to homes and stuff it is only when there

is too much violence in the house and where the person would never be cared for. In [town] I have known a family where there was lot of violence in the house and the old woman who was there that had some kind of a problem where she was squashed up into the bed and her legs pulled up and no one there to clean her and no one there to look after her at all. And the worst thing is, when outsiders came, the old women would show her leg to outsiders as if there was something to inspect. This is the horrible situation that goes within the family and, in that case, she would have been better off in the home. *(Interview for Divya Chadha's PhD)*

In other situations, it may be that the person with dementia is abusing the carer, possibly due to misunderstanding brought about by dementia-related confusion. One of our interviewees lived alone with her husband, who was considerably older than herself. The couple's two sons visited regularly but the husband, who no longer recognized them, thought his wife was improperly entertaining them. She cared for her husband for ten years but came to a breaking point due to his aggressive behaviour.

> Then he started being suspicious of my sons, thinking they are my boyfriends and he said, 'Don't you feel ashamed, one comes when the other goes,' because they didn't turn up at the same time. They used to come after one another. He said, 'Don't you feel ashamed with these men coming after one another, you should die with the embarrassment you bring onto me.' Then he started getting very violent, he didn't hit me but shouted, and bawling and stuff like that. Then slowly I said to [social worker], 'You have to do something.' He said, 'The only thing you can do is send him to a home.' That's when we sent him into a home. *(Interview for Caregiving HOPE)*

In addition to situations of abuse, other issues which can be triggers for nursing home care are related to particular care needs. Managing incontinence, for example, can be very hard for some people, the need to lift someone can cause difficulties, and some families may feel out of depth in providing end-of-life care.

> **POINT FOR PRACTICE: CONSIDER SAFEGUARDING ISSUES**
>
> The examples above raise the importance of awareness of the possibility of abuse, which can often be a hidden problem. It is vital that professionals do not let assumptions that care at home is 'a good thing' cloud their ability to be open to signs of mistreatment. It is also important to be aware that it can be either the person with dementia who is being mistreated or the carer who may be suffering at the hands of the individual with dementia. Opening up a non-judgemental conversation and offering culturally suitable and sanctioned support can be steps to exploring and improving a situation. Safeguarding procedures, as dictated by the Care Act (2014), would have to be followed if indicated, so all staff need to be aware of these.

Societal and generational changes

There are some indications that people from minority ethnic communities may be gradually moving away from family-centred care, as living situations and ways of life of successive generations in the UK evolve (see Chapter 5, section on cultural and religious influences on family care). Where there are smaller, more dispersed families and there is a need for all working-age members of a household to go out to work, care cannot be shared among siblings as it would have been within an extensive available local family network. The care situation then becomes more like that of many White British families where care tends to fall on a spouse, a single local daughter or the next closest relative. One of our research participants of South Asian ethnicity expresses this point. He had siblings he thought he could count on to share care but recognized this would not be the case in all families:

> I mean if it comes to it, I don't know, as a family we would have some kind of meeting, but I think, I think we could all look after her. I don't think, I don't think she'd need to go to a care home, I

personally don't think she would need it. I personally think that my sisters wouldn't think that, my brothers wouldn't think it. You know, I mean, if you're on your own I can understand, you know, you do need help, if you've got somebody who's not looking after you, you're on your own, then I think a care home's better with people, you know, looking after you, and you've got people, sort of, the age groups and all that, and you have a routine there, whatever. *(Interview for Caregiving HOPE)*

An article in *The Guardian* on the growing number of South Asian care home places in 2011 reinforced that changes may be due to these pragmatic alterations in families' way of life, The journalist, Sarfraz Manzoor (2011), noted that residents in the care home he visited tended to be Indian, middle class and have only one or two children. This is echoed in an interview from the Caregiving HOPE study where a daughter was asked if she had considered care home placement and said:

No, not, I mean I know that it exists, I know more and more people are sending their parents to care homes, you know, especially the people that are actually well educated and, um, you know, they don't have time for their parents, you know, they'd rather [just] sit. *(Interview for Caregiving HOPE)*

In addition to changing lifestyles, the assimilation of British majority values by second and subsequent generation British people of minority ethnicities may be influencing attitudes to care. This is a process often referred to as acculturation (Ward, 2008) and is well expressed here by one of Divya Chadha's PhD participants of South Asian ethnicity who is critical of the changes he sees in some others in his community.

People who were living in India and Pakistan would look after the person themselves. They would never think of sending them anywhere. When they come to the West, they find the comfort, the enjoyment of the world and that life is forever, want to enjoy, like paradise on Earth. And a mother or a father becomes a burden to them and even though they don't want to think like that but sub-consciously they are thinking like that. And when the time comes they think, oh my father is old, he will be better off in a home. He will be fooled into believing that his father is better off in a home. *(Interview for Divya Chadha's PhD)*

In some families this may lead to differences between generations' views of the best place for an older person with advanced dementia to be cared for, with the older generation holding the traditional view and the children thinking of care home placement as the best solution.

> Because my dad's like, he's, he's really reluctant to doing it. Because for me, um, 'cause I've already obviously thought about it. So the way I've thought about it is that we still have her at home up until the point where she probably doesn't know where home is because she doesn't recognize it. So if we put her into a care home at that point it wouldn't really matter 'cause she wouldn't know where home is really but, whatever, that's way in the future then, you know. *(Interview for Caregiving HOPE)*

This almost casual assertion that it would not matter to put their mum in a care home once she is unable to recognize her family contrasts with the interviewee's report of her dad's feelings on the subject:

> My dad says he's just scared that, she may not, like she may get really frustrated there, that she may believe that we ditched her. So, he doesn't want her to think that, like, we ditched her and then he, he, he thinks that 'Oh, she's just gonna do whatever it takes, just for her just to, like, get out' and that will be really dangerous for her... And then, yeah, so he just, he's just thinking that she may not even last a week in a care home, and then if anything happens he's just like, he doesn't want to have that blame you know. *(Interview for Caregiving HOPE)*

> **POINT FOR PRACTICE: THE IMPORTANCE OF WORKING WITH FAMILIES**
> In line with familism (see Chapter 5), many minority ethnic families may take a family decision about care arrangements. However, as illustrated above, there may be differences between family members that need to be addressed to jointly agree on the way forward. As such, having skills in family work, and having some appreciation for the power structures in different minority ethnic communities, can be important for health and social care staff.

Coping with stigma

When families do move a relative to a care home, they frequently face stigma from their extended family or from the community for breaking the usual conventions (see Table 6.1). The presence of this stigma strengthens the reluctance of families to use care homes.

Table 6.1: Examples of external pressures to continue to care at home

Pressure from the wider family	What I took issue with is where people like brothers-in-law who are from Pakistan, they are the ones that would still have those traditional views and would say, 'What are you doing, that's haram, you shouldn't be doing that to your mum, this that and the other.' I would be like 'You don't know what you're talking about, if you spent 24 hours in our shoes, then you'll understand.' So I found them to be more judgemental than the direct family. That's the issue, that's something that needs to be tackled, it's not the inner family, it's the extended. (Caregiving HOPE)
Pressure from the wider society or community	Researcher: Did you say it was an obligation to provide care? Participant: Obligation and duty. As a Muslim and as a son to look after the parents no matter what. The community judges individuals on that, rightly or wrongly, they do. (Caregiving HOPE)

Some families respond to community stigma by trying to find ways to ignore judgemental comments from others. The woman we quoted above, who had placed her husband in a care home due to his abusive behaviour towards her, spoke of the way others in the community gossiped about her:

> Even now they sometimes say, 'She's kicked her husband out, and she's now enjoying herself on her own at home.' They used to say a lot in the beginning, I just ignore it now so they [say it] less and less now. *(Interview for Caregiving HOPE)*

Going against convention often leaves family members feeling guilty about their decision. Even though this woman felt her decision was necessary, she still felt to blame if ever her husband seemed low:

> Sometimes when I go visit him now, if he's very down, he just sleeps and he doesn't respond, then I'm very upset until the next visit, thinking, 'What have I done to him! God is punishing me!' When I was ill, I thought that was the way of God to punish me and people said, 'No, he's in good hands. He's getting looked after better than when he was here' ...but in my inner heart I think I punished him. *(Interview for Caregiving HOPE)*

In cases where faith is involved, it may be possible to provide a religious interpretation or blessing to show that moving to a care home is acceptable and virtuous. For example, one man of Pakistani Muslim background, in the Caregiving HOPE study, had made the difficult decision to place his mother in a nursing home. He sought the blessing of an imam (Islamic scholar) and he felt comforted by the thought that he could quote this to show he was not being un-Islamic if he was criticized by those in his community. He said:

> So, putting my mum in a care home, so again I needed permission from the Imam. Can I seek help, help for respite as a Muslim? He said they could hear mum, because they're next-door neighbours.

She needs 24/7 care so, yes, you are permitted to do that. So the fact that he's given the blessings to do it, I'm still conscious of what the community will think...because then I could say to whoever, 'What are you talking about? I've asked, not just an imam or a hafiz, a mufti, and he said, "Yes according to hadith, yes, you are allowed to seek help."' *(Interview for Caregiving HOPE)*

> **POINT FOR PRACTICE: SUPPORT FAMILY MEMBERS TO ADJUST IF A RELATIVE MOVES TO A CARE HOME**
> Health and social care professionals need to be aware of the potential isolation and guilt that many family members feel if their relative with dementia has moved to live-in care. Taking steps to support people to manage such feelings and providing links to other carers in similar positions may be helpful.

Different family configurations

Many South Asian communities in the UK have close ties with their extended family and community even if life is changing across generations. However, many immigrants may have left their wider family in their country of origin and be relatively isolated in the UK. Others may not have children to rely on. Further, not all minority ethnic cultures are built around family closeness.

UK Government (2024) figures show how common it is for older White British people to live in an 'all pensioner' household or alone. Across 'all pensioner households', 98% are White British, 1.6% are Asian and 0.6% are Black. Fifteen per cent of all White British households are made up of an older person who lives alone, compared with 7% of Black households, 5% of mixed and 4% of Asian households. Living alone makes the likelihood of moving into a care home 20 times higher than it is for someone living in a household with others (Banerjee *et al.*, 2003), so this implies that more White British people are vulnerable from this point of view, but numbers in the Black population are also quite significant.

> **POINT FOR PRACTICE: DON'T MAKE ASSUMPTIONS AROUND SUPPORT – ASK ABOUT SUPPORT NETWORKS**
>
> It is important not to make assumptions around circumstances on the basis of ethnicity, given that increasing numbers across all ethnic groups in the UK are living in one- or two-person households. When it comes to understanding a person's living situation, everyone needs to be considered as an individual, so for each and every person, we need to ask what support they have available to them and whether or not there are family members or friends they can rely on for practical support.

Living in a care home

In this section, we present some figures about how many people from minority ethnic groups live in care homes and then consider key issues of importance (communication, food, social connections and activities, faith and racism) in providing appropriate care for people of diverse ethnicities. For each issue we give relevant contextual information and put forward some points for practice.

Numbers of people from minority ethnic communities who live in care homes

In the White British population, almost two out of every three people with dementia live in the community and about a third in a care home (Prince et al., 2014). There is very little information on how many people with dementia from minority ethnic backgrounds live in care homes. However, many care homes do have residents with non-White British cultural backgrounds. Two surveys have both found that about one in three care homes reported diversity among their residents. A postal survey (Badger et al., 2012) in an unspecified region of the UK found a third of 101 care homes had at least one resident from a minority ethnic background. A further survey of 86 English care homes found more than a third (38%) had at least one resident whose first language was not English (Cooper *et al.*, 2018). Of over 1000 care home residents in the second survey, one in every 20 (5%) spoke English as a second language

These figures show that it is not rare for care homes to have residents from minority ethnic populations and raise the question of how adequately care homes provide for diverse residents. It has been observed that those from minority ethnic backgrounds in care homes are younger, and more likely to be male, have dementia and incontinence and be more dependent than those from White British backgrounds (Milne & Smith, 2015).

Culturally specific care homes

Some care homes cater specifically for particular ethnic communities. However, at present there are few such homes. The Jewish community is an exception, with the charity Jewish Care listing 50 Jewish care homes across the UK run by itself and others. Other ethnicity-specific care homes are rare but may be increasing. For example, Manchester City Council in 2014 had care homes that specialized in provision for the Polish, Slovenian and Asian communities as well as some that had a high percentage of Chinese or Caribbean residents. The difference culturally competent care can make to a person feeling at home cannot be over-emphasized. One report gives an example of an older person of Chinese origin who moved 100 miles away from the son she used to live with so that she could live in specialist Chinese sheltered housing with a care facility (Manthorpe *et al.*, 2010). The report states:

> She had previously lived with her son but was getting increasingly isolated as he was at work all day, compounded by the effects of her long-term health conditions and a recent stroke. She had been on the waiting list for over a year before there was a vacancy. The support she valued was the language, the food and the general atmosphere, just being able to watch a game of Mah-jong now she could no longer play herself.

Living in a 'generic' care home

Care homes that are not culturally specific but which take residents from diverse backgrounds face challenges of finding out about culturally related needs and finding ways to meet them. There are few published first-hand or observational accounts of what life is like for people with dementia who live in care homes but interviews with relatives and care home staff, as well as statistical data, give a picture of what is important (Badger *et al.*, 2012). Key issues identified by Badger's study included food, social connections and activities, communication, faith and racism.

We address each of these below. In the quote below (which we chose also as an opening quote for this chapter), a family member describes what was important to him in looking for a suitable care home for his mother and what happened when a home was not culturally competent:

> Either staff being from the same culture, religion or ethnicity or residents from that background, so that at least staff are familiar with the culture and religion. The quality of care, CQC reports, in terms of how good they are; how aware they are of the issues, so are they saying the right things: 'Yeah, yeah, we know about Islam, we know about halal.' Those kind of right words, you just get that feeling. We had to get the closest thing, there wasn't anything that ticked all the boxes.
>
> Wherever we went there wasn't a single person that was Pakistani, Asian, Muslim, whatever. So that's an issue because they didn't really understand her needs, cultural, dietary, religious and so on. We found one place, and within one day we got a call from the place saying, 'We can't cope with your mum's needs, can you take her? We can't cope with her needs, she's disturbing the other residents, can you take her home?' *(Interview for Caregiving HOPE)*

PERSONAL CARE

An issue not identified by research but which is important in practice is personal care, including washing, skincare, grooming and dressing, which all have a cultural angle. Dark skin, for example, may benefit from daily moisturiser and the person may have a particular type that is preferred. A Black person's hair may not need daily combing if there are braids in place but when hair is combed it will require an Afro-style comb not a fine-toothed English comb. There may also be cultural aspects to toilet use, washing, who should assist in relation to gender and what sort of clothing should be worn.

> **POINT FOR PRACTICE: GETTING PERSONAL CARE RIGHT**
> Getting small aspects of personal care right may make all the difference to someone feeling at home. This means that it is very important to find out the detail of each individual's former routines, likes and dislikes. This can be done using a 'This is me' style form (see Alzheimer's Society, 2021).

FOOD
Most people take comfort and delight in food and drinks for their own sake as well as for the social side of mealtimes. In care homes, mealtimes are prominent events, especially as residents often cannot do the other things that generally mark out time. However, compared with living at home, people in care homes have little choice over who they eat with, and when, what and how they eat. Those with advanced dementia can be doubly disadvantaged as their sense of taste may be affected by dementia and their ability to chew and swallow food may be impaired, affecting the quality of their experience.

Food preferences and habits are strongly influenced by culture and, for some, by religion. Culture influences what is eaten and routines, expected mealtimes and ways of eating. For religious reasons, food may need to be kosher, halal or vegan, or certain meats may need to be avoided. In a survey of nursing home managers, some felt training in specific ways of catering could enable care homes to provide appropriate food, whereas others cited how helpful it was when relatives were able to bring food in (Badger *et al.*, 2012).

> **POINT FOR PRACTICE: INDIVIDUAL FOOD PREFERENCES**
>
> In line with person-centred care, to help people with advanced dementia feel at home, it is important to know about their food preferences and, if possible, to find out about the flavours and tastes from their childhood. Rather than make cultural generalizations, finding out about each person is important, as stated by a care home manager:
>
> > I've learned from bitter experience that one must not rule out the fact that because somebody comes from a certain ethnic background, they may not always want to eat the kind of food that their families or their community do. (Heather, care home manager; Manthorpe et al., 2010)

As there are limits to what a care home is able to provide, enabling relatives to bring food, alongside instructing them about any issues necessary to reduce risk, can help a resident have that sense of something familiar. When relatives bring in food, it is important to let staff and other residents know and respond if others are unhappy or intolerant (Manthorpe et al., 2010). Another possibility is for staff to organize for a resident to go out to an ethnically based lunch club where the person can have a taste of home (Manthorpe et al., 2010).

SOCIAL CONNECTION AND ACTIVITIES

It has been known for a long time that having something meaningful to do is helpful for mental health. This applies also to those living with dementia. As impairment increases, it can be hard to find things a person is capable of, but most care homes have activities coordinators who specialize in finding suitable activities.

ACTIVITY 6.1: IDENTIFYING CULTURALLY SUITABLE ACTIVITIES

Below, we have listed some activities that are used in care homes. In this exercise, think about whether each would be familiar to a White British 75-year-old and a 75-year-old from a South Asian background. Then consider whether each would need to be adapted in some way, and suggest some ideas for adaptation.

Activity	How familiar to a White British 75-year-old?	How familiar to a South Asian 75-year-old?	How much adaptation for a 75-year-old from a South Asian background?	How could it be adapted?
Reminiscence about childhood and earlier life				
Listening to chart music of the 1960s				
Making collages				
Knitting				
Throwing a ball				

cont.

Activity	How familiar to a White British 75-year-old?	How familiar to a South Asian 75-year-old?	How much adaptation for a 75-year-old from a South Asian background?	How could it be adapted?
Gardening				
Kneading dough				
Tai chi				
Hand massage				
Aromatherapy				

COMMUNICATION

A common experience for minority ethnic residents is to be the only person of their background in their care home. One survey of 86 care homes found that, across the 13 homes where there were South Asian residents, there was only one South Asian resident in each, and in eight of the 14 care homes with Black residents, there was only person who was Black (Badger *et al.*, 2012). This can be an isolating experience. Even where a home specializes in provision for a particular community, it is important to remember that diversity exists in every population. One older retired actor of Pakistani origin, living in a specialist home for the South Asian community where most residents were of Indian origin, told *The Guardian* journalist Sarfraz Manzoor, 'I have no friends here so I am not happy: the Gujaratis keep themselves to themselves; the Patels do the same. I wish there were more Pakistanis here' (Manzoor, 2011).

Isolation can be particularly acute where language prevents communication. The fear of being isolated due to language barriers may deter use of care homes (Mold, Fitzpatrick & Roberts, 2005). Of the 86 homes in Cooper *et al.*'s (2018) study, 23 had only one resident who spoke English as a second language. In advanced dementia, people may revert to the language of their childhood, leaving them unable to easily communicate their needs or understand what staff are saying to them. Where people who cannot communicate are placed in care, their communication difficulties may lead to distress and agitated or aggressive behaviour. One study found a significant link between residents having English as a second language and higher levels of agitation and disturbed behaviour (Cooper *et al.*, 2018). The most plausible explanation is that where people with dementia do not understand what is happening and become frustrated or distressed, their unmet needs are expressed through their actions. The staff interviewed by Cooper *et al.* held the view that language barriers not only increased residents' agitation but were also a cause of distress to staff and residents alike.

> **POINT FOR PRACTICE: COMMUNICATION NEEDS**
> It is important for care staff to try and find ways of communicating, whether by language or non-verbally (Cooper *et al.*, 2018). A number of approaches have been suggested and are shown in Table 6.2.

Table 6.2: Approaches to improving communication between staff and care home residents who do not speak fluent English

- Homes may be able to employ staff who understand and speak the language in question.

- Homes may be able to locate a volunteer or a member of staff at a neighbouring care home. Manthorpe *et al.* (2010) give examples of calls being put out by a local authority to care homes in their area, to find people with specific language skills.

- Residents who are usually non-verbal may speak a few words or phrases in their mother tongue which may be significant. A focus on finding out what the resident is saying can be helpful.

- Family members may be willing to make sound recordings of key messages related to care or comfort that can be played for a resident (Badger *et al.*, 2012). As Badger points out, although this may be helpful for routine day-to-day care, it cannot meet needs in emergencies. A further major disadvantage is that this only supports one-way communication from staff to residents and may not help residents to make their views known.

- Families may be able to act as interpreters, although they are not always there and, as key intermediaries with beliefs and opinions of their own, they may sometimes change the messages as they translate (Badger *et al.*, 2012).

- Pictures of common communication objects can be helpful, including for meal and clothing choices.

- Gaining understanding from family members of the person's body language and the ways they would usually find solace if distressed can enable staff to understand and respond to distress. Where one person may express distress through agitation and restlessness, another may express this through becoming quiet and withdrawn. Equally, one person may feel more secure and calm if a member of staff brushes her hair or holds her hand, whereas for another, it might be that hugging a favourite object is more helpful.

Overall, it feels as if there is no substitute for being with others who share your own language but where this is not the case, there are alternatives that can be tried.

FAITH AND RELIGION

As noted elsewhere, faith is a strong backdrop to many people's lives, not least for those in minority ethnic communities. The

UK has strong Christian traditions. In keeping with this, nine in ten care home managers in Badger *et al.*'s (2012) survey reported having a good or very good understanding of Christianity. Even here, however, there are different denominations and ways of worship that benefit from cultural understanding. The daughter of a woman of African-Caribbean origin living in care illustrated this in relation to her mother's care:

> We actually found a home that was run by a Jamaican nurse, it had a lot of Caribbeans in it anyway. She thought it was her home. She only lasted one day in a home that wasn't culturally competent, she fought them there as well. When we found this one, she was happy there. They had their church services, people came in. *('Raeni', interviewed for Saba Shaiq's PhD)*

Raeni went on to describe the way her father was able to help another distressed resident, using his approach to Christianity:

> Particularly black people, they look out for each other. My father even said on one occasion there was an elder. They call the elders 'mother', and she was 'Mother [name]'. She had signs of dementia and she was being quite aggressive to her daughter. She would lock herself in the room. ... They were having a prayer meeting that day, and he said, in the end, he knocked on the door and asked her to come and join them and they prayed for her. She came to faith quite late in life that woman, but he said after that prayer, she came back to a normal mind and they didn't have any problems until she died. *('Raeni', interviewed for Saba Shafiq's PhD)*

This shows the sense of mutual understanding and support within this Black community and that this woman's aggressive behaviour was seen as having been soothed by prayer with her peers.

Where the religion is not a denomination of Christianity but is a non-Christian religion there will be many points of difference that need to be appreciated to provide appropriate care. In Badger *et al.*'s (2012) survey, under half of home managers felt they had a good or very good understanding of other religions. This has significant implications for supporting spiritual needs, religious observations and practices.

> **POINT FOR PRACTICE: BE RESPECTFULLY CURIOUS ABOUT RELIGION**
>
> Although it is not possible to know about all religions in depth, staff should not hesitate to be respectfully curious. Conversations with family, colleagues, chaplains and religious figures (priests, imams and so on) may be helpful. While it may be hard to provide fully for spiritual needs in care homes that are largely secular and have diverse staff, some small changes could be easy to implement. A doctoral study conducted at our Centre for Applied Dementia Studies in Bradford (Collins, 2020), for example, found that many older White British residents had been used to saying grace (i.e., making a short religious prayer) before meals to be thankful to God for their food – a practice that would be easy for staff to introduce for those who need it.

RACISM

A final issue to mention that can arise in the care home setting where there are diverse residents is that of people from ethnic minorities being the object of racism. There is little mention of overt racism in published papers but there is evidence of ignorance about cultural issues and anecdotal evidence of imposition of stereotypes and intolerance of difference, for example in relation to preferred foods.

As we saw earlier in this chapter, experiences of racism may deter people from minority ethnic backgrounds from considering the use of care homes, or may lead to them being very wary. One African-Caribbean interviewee described how the family were so concerned about possible mistreatment that they set up a visiting rota and dropped into the mother's care home unannounced so they could check up on the quality of care.

I didn't want to put her in a situation where she was mistreated, and we've put her there. That's one of the reasons why we would go every single day, even if I say that I would go in the morning then somebody else would go in the afternoon, so we kept it consistent. We wouldn't even stick to certain times. We'd literally just go in there, so the staff didn't know when to expect us just to keep them on their toes as well. *(Interviewed by Saba Shafiq)*

ACTIVITY 6.2: IDENTIFYING AND ACTING ON CULTURALLY RELATED ISSUES

A group of people living with dementia from University of Bradford worked with us to develop short scenarios that captured their experiences of care (Capstick *et al.*, 2021). Read the scenario below and look out for issues related to culture. Considering Ella, what issues can you identify? Suggest at least two things that could be done to improve her situation.

After you have thought about your suggestions, have a look at our ideas at the end of the chapter.

It is 11am and Christine and Ella, both women living with dementia, are sitting next to each other in the lounge of the care home. It's a quiet day, and no one else is sitting nearby. For most of the following hour Christine seems to be having a conversation with someone who isn't actually there. At times, she replies to herself in a different, deeper tone of voice, and she often mentions someone called Bob. She talks mainly about a time when she was injured and had to go to hospital. Her hearing aid is in upside down.

Ella has a worried look. She doesn't talk much, but every now and then she will try to start a conversation with Christine by asking a polite question, such as 'When did that happen?' Whenever she does this Christine's face takes on an angry expression and she replies to Ella in a harsh voice, telling her off. Ella looks as though she is about to cry. A passing member of staff says, 'Play nicely, girls.' Ella says that she wants to go home, and that everything was better back home, when she used to help out at the mission.

At 12 o'clock another member of staff tells Christine and Ella that they can have either shepherd's pie or fish and chips for lunch. 'You don't like fish,' she tells Ella. Ella replies, 'I do like fish. I like saltfish. I just don't like your white fish.'

Diversity among staff: Asset or problem?

One interesting issue regarding care home care is how to best use the potential asset of the diversity among staff. As with many low-pay sectors of the economy, many people who work in care homes are from outside the UK. Badger *et al.*'s (2012) survey found that 95% of care homes had minority ethnic staff; almost three-quarters (73%) had staff of South Asian ethnicity and almost two-thirds (64%) had staff who identified as Black. Care home managers reported that having immigrant staff, especially if their English is accented or poor, could lead to misunderstandings between staff and residents and provoke racist comments from White British residents (Manthorpe *et al.*, 2018). It can also result in factions, cliques and conflicts among staff (Manthorpe *et al.*, 2018). On the other hand, Badger and colleagues found that many care home managers perceived staff diversity as a strength as they were able to draw on the cultural knowledge of staff members as well as their language skills to meet the needs of residents from similar backgrounds.

Steps towards culturally appropriate care for minority ethnic residents

Mold, Fitzpatrick and Roberts (2005), in the conclusions of their international review of research about 'ethnic elders' in care homes, concluded that collaborations and training are two essentials needed to ensure culturally appropriate care home care.

First, they suggested a need for greater collaboration between the third sector, the independent care home sector and the government. This is echoed by Manthorpe *et al.* (2010), who pointed out the two-way advantages that would come from closer partnerships. Working together could bring the specialist cultural knowledge of minority ethnic organizations to the attention of care staff and enable staff from minority ethnic organizations to learn about specialist aspects of dementia care.

Second, Mold, Fitzpatrick and Roberts (2005) proposed that research-informed training and education would raise the awareness of care home staff. Manthorpe *et al.* (2010) found that social care staff had received training about cultural aspects of food, faith and death rituals but also needed training around how to promote well-being. Cooper *et al.* (2018) highlighted that communication is essential to care well for people living with dementia. They suggest staff learning key words, and use of technology could help.

There remains a question about how well staff manage to act on training, as reported by one of the interviewees in the Caregiving HOPE study:

> The staff are also I would say quite frankly clueless, don't know if they've gone through any equality and diversity training, they are clueless, so I ended up in one place educating them about halal, about how they shouldn't contaminate the meat, so they had 2 shelves then, they had halal at the top and non halal at bottom, so there was no cross-contamination, things like that. *(Interview for Caregiving HOPE)*

> **POINT FOR PRACTICE: KEEPING ETHNICITY ON THE AGENDA**
> When was the last time you discussed cultural aspects of care in relation to care for someone living with dementia? Other pressing aspects of care may push cultural considerations down the agenda, so it may be helpful for staff to have routine opportunities to reflect explicitly on cultural aspects of care for their residents, in resident reviews, supervision or staff meetings.

Conclusion

There is limited research into use of care homes by people from minority ethnic backgrounds. However, it is clear that we must move beyond the assumption that 'they look after their own'. A significant and probably increasing number of people with advanced dementia from minority ethnic groups are moving into care, yet this still carries stigma and it remains hard to find culturally appropriate care for people from minority ethnic communities. In this chapter, we have highlighted key issues to consider in improving care so it provides for the diversity of the population and can meet the needs of people of all ethnicities. Whether people are living at home or in care, dementia is a progressive condition that shortens life. In the next chapter, we address issues around end of life and bereavement of a family member with dementia.

> **REFLECTIONS ON ACTIVITY 6.2**
> The interaction between Ella and Christine is strained but they are left with each other for an hour without staff taking more than passing notice. We can see hints that Ella grew up in the Caribbean. One comes from her statement that she used to help out 'at the mission', a term often used to describe a Caribbean religion-based community centre. It sounds as if she is longing to be back in that familiar environment. Another is related to her statement that she likes saltfish, which is not usually part of a White British diet but is common in the Caribbean.
>
> Considering this, staff could offer Ella a reminiscence box or a set of pictures related to life in the Caribbean which would give her a meaningful activity that connects with her identity. Staff could try and find out what music Ella used to listen to – perhaps she listened to praise music, ska or reggae. She could have a personalized playlist to listen to. Thinking of her comment on 'your white fish', it seems Ella is missing the familiar foods of her earlier life. Perhaps staff could find out more about her favourite foods and see if there are any she could be offered that would provide comfort and familiarity.

Chapter 7

Advance Care Planning, End of Life and Bereavement

My message to the Asian community is, we don't have to be heroes like I attempted to be and do everything on our own. There is some really good support out there. We shouldn't be ashamed to take that support out there.

(SUKHNINDER PANESAR, HEAD OF LAW, WOLVERHAMPTON UNIVERSITY; HYATT, 2019)

Introduction

This final chapter looks at issues around the end of life of people of minority ethnicities living with dementia. The chapter is divided into four sections.

- The first section sets the scene with definitions, facts and figures.
- The second section looks at ways people living with dementia can make their views and wishes about how they would like to be cared for known in advance.
- In the third section, we look at best practice in end-of-life care for people from minority ethnicities.
- In the fourth section, we think about the needs of family members who are bereaved of someone with dementia.

Definitions, facts and figures
Dementia as a terminal illness

Dementia is considered to be a *terminal disease* because it is life-shortening. Put bluntly, dementia is an incurable condition which gets worse over time and is a leading cause of death. The fact that people can have many years of living reasonably well with dementia after diagnosis may contribute to the perception that it is not a terminal condition. However, without taking this on board, it is all too easy to delay the process of planning for future care.

People live, on average, between one and eight and a half years after a diagnosis of dementia, but there is a lot of variability (Brodaty, Seeher & Gibson, 2012). The older you are at diagnosis the shorter your survival time (Brodaty, Seeher & Gibson, 2012). This has implications for people from minority ethnic backgrounds, who tend to seek a diagnosis later in the dementia trajectory, so they will have fewer years ahead of them by the time they are diagnosed. We do not have a lot of direct knowledge about how ethnicity influences life expectancy in dementia. However, one international review summarized 22 studies comparing mortality after diagnosis across at least two ethnic samples (Co *et al.*, 2021). Most of the research had been conducted in the US and just three studies had been carried out in the UK, but Co and colleagues concluded that:

- mortality risk for people with dementia is lower in US Black/African American and Hispanic/Latino populations
- the pattern of lower mortality risk in older non-White populations with dementia is also present in the UK.

A similar pattern was found when Co and colleagues looked at the records of one large London Trust over a ten-year period, finding that compared to the White British, risk of death was lower in White Irish, Black Caribbean, Black African and South Asian ethnicities (Co *et al.*, 2023). There is no clear explanation for this at the present time but there is some evidence that it may only be true of first-generation migrants, in which case it may be explained by the hypothesis that those who choose to emigrate are hardier and healthier than those who remain at home (Co *et al.*, 2023).

Palliative and end-of-life care

NHS England defines palliative care as:

> an approach that improves the quality of life of patients and their families facing the problems associated with life-threatening or life-limiting illness, through the prevention and relief of suffering by means of early identification and impeccable assessment and treatment of pain and other problems, physical, psychosocial and spiritual. *(NHS England, 2022)*

Palliative care aims to be holistic, with a focus on quality of life for people and their families. The approach originally developed in cancer care but is applicable for all serious illnesses that cannot be cured. It can be used at any point from diagnosis onwards.

End-of-life care is care provided towards the end of life, often defined as the last year, although sometimes it refers to the last weeks or days of life. It is estimated that 30 per cent of people aged 65 or over will die with dementia (Brayne *et al.*, 2006), so end-of-life care is relevant to dementia care. This chapter is more concerned with end-of-life than palliative care, but where the two have been grouped together by researchers or practitioners, we have used the term 'palliative and end-of-life care'.

Dementia is mentioned just once in the *statutory guidance on palliative and end of life care for integrated care boards* (NHS England, 2022). The guidance says that integrated care boards should work in partnership with system-level networks, including those focused on dementia, to ensure the delivery of high quality personalised Palliative and End of Life Care for everyone, in all care settings. How accessible palliative and end-of-life care are for people living with dementia and their families, especially for those from minority ethnic groups, and how the approaches need to be adapted to be appropriate, will be addressed in the third section of this chapter.

Advance care planning

Advance care planning is the process of thinking ahead to influence the care you will receive at the end of life or from a point when you lose cognitive capacity to make your views known or to give consent to important decisions. There are different elements of advance care planning that have different meanings and legal statuses. These are complex and we only cover them very briefly here:

- *Advance statements* give a person's wishes, preferences, beliefs and values about their future care. They have to be taken into account by those responsible for care but are not legally binding (National Council for Palliative Care and National End of Life Care Programme, 2013, p.5).
- *An advance decision to refuse treatment (ADRT)* is used to express a wish not to have specific interventions that could sustain life but which the person would rather avoid. These are legally binding.
- *Do not attempt cardiopulmonary resuscitation* orders, often referred to as DNACPRs or DNRs (do not resuscitate), are, as the name implies, orders not to attempt to restart a person's heart should it stop beating. A doctor or medical team can also place a DNR order on medical notes. They should inform the person unless they think doing so will cause the person harm; in other words, doctors can decide this for you and do not have to tell you about it.

There is further information and guidance available about this complex area of terminology on NHS sites, for example:

- www.nhs.uk/conditions/end-of-life-care/planning-ahead/why-plan-ahead
- www.england.nhs.uk/improvement-hub/wp-content/uploads/sites/44/2017/11/Advance-Decisions-to-Refuse-Treatment-Guide.pdf
- www.nhs.uk/conditions/do-not-attempt-cardiopulmonary-resuscitation-dnacpr-decisions

Why do advance care planning?

Both living with advanced dementia and dying involve loss of control and high levels of dependence on others. So advance care planning can be valuable in relation to advanced dementia care as well as in relation to end of life. The process gives people the chance to discover and to inform others about what they want for themselves. Making their wishes known helps to ensure the best quality of life at end of life.

A key consideration in advance care planning is the preferred balance between interventions and palliative care. Some people want to prolong life and have treatment, for example with resuscitation and intravenous antibiotics, while others would prefer to die sooner without 'aggressive' intervention. Using advance care planning, these views can be made known. People can also voice other preferences, for example a person could specify that they want to avoid admission to an acute hospital or, if a person has a strong view that they would prefer to have a formal carer rather than have a daughter feel over-burdened, this could equally be expressed.

Advance care planning is especially relevant in dementia because at advanced stages people are not in a position to communicate their wishes easily. Making care decisions can be a heavy burden for family and care staff if they have to guess what the person would have wished to happen. Illustrating that the relative and the 'patient' may have different points of view, one US study interviewed people with cancer at end of life and their next-of-kin. They found disagreement between the patient and the next-of-kin among those without advance statements in relation to cardiopulmonary resuscitation in 46% of the dyads and mechanical ventilation in 50% (Phipps *et al.*, 2003).

People often assume they will be able to rely on their next-of-kin to make decisions for them if they are not able to voice what they want but if there has been no advance statement and no one has been appointed as a lasting power of attorney, then the next-of-kin does not have the last say on healthcare decisions. Instead, these rest with the medical staff, who have to judge what is in the person's best interests.

Barriers to advance care planning

In a review of advance care planning in dementia, the authors found only three articles reporting original research from the UK or Europe (Mountford, Dening & Green, 2024). They summarize general barriers to advance care planning in dementia. One in particular is that it is hard to choose the right moment. It may feel too soon after diagnosis, when there is an emphasis on living well, but if left too long, the person may lose capacity to voice their views.

Although Mountford, Dening and Green (2024) did not find any British or European studies focused on minority ethnic populations, we can surmise that there are issues to keep in mind:

- *Lack of dementia awareness and delayed diagnosis:* Later diagnosis reduces opportunities for advance care planning. More people from minority ethnic communities may be diagnosed at a point where their cognitive impairment is too great for them to join in advance care planning discussions (Dlamini, 2021).

- *Cultural values:* It has been suggested that advance care planning is rooted in western values that emphasize autonomy and individual rights. These values may not be strongly present in other cultures (Kagawa-Singer & Blackhall, 2001). In more interdependent cultures, individuals may feel it is selfish to push forward their own wishes, so this can be a barrier to advance planning.

    Death is a taboo subject in many cultures. We are used to euphemisms, such as talking about someone 'passing' rather than 'dying' to avoid causing discomfort to ourselves and others. Discussing death and dying may be taboo for people from some minority ethnic backgrounds, especially if there are superstitious beliefs that by talking about dying, a person might make it more likely.

- *Religious beliefs:* Many people of faith feel they should not fear death and, indeed, religion can lessen fears of death (Jong *et al.*, 2017). Some religions may encourage people to accept that God is in charge and knows best, so struggling to gain personal control over death might seem to be contrary to God's will. As religious belief tends to be stronger among ethnic minority populations in the UK, this probably means more people from these communities will feel it is not appropriate to discuss end of life than is the case for the indigenous White British.

- *Trust in services:* As noted in earlier chapters, people from ethnic minorities may not readily trust officialdom, so committing advance wishes to paper in a statement or a directive might be avoided in case it is somehow misused.

- *Legal frameworks:* Older immigrants to the UK may have little knowledge of legal frameworks. It is often assumed that a next-of-kin will be able to make appropriate decisions and the person may not appreciate that setting up a lasting power of attorney for health and welfare is necessary to ensure this.

- *Staff assumptions:* Staff may avoid talking with people with dementia from minority ethnic backgrounds about advance care planning, assuming that this would be uncomfortable, offensive or not appropriate. Staff may lack competence or confidence to raise the issues. This may be exacerbated by the organizational divide between mental health services (where most people with dementia receive care) and physical health services (where palliative and end-of-life care teams are based). Staff in palliative care teams may have more experience in opening up these sensitive conversations.

A recent PhD study (Dlamini, 2021) on views of end-of-life care of African and Caribbean people with dementia in the UK found that religious and cultural pressures made participants suffer in silence, as they felt they should have faith in God rather than make any plans of their own. However, the findings also showed that people wished to prioritize quality of life at the end of life, so this potentially could open a door to discussion.

How to address advance care planning with people from minority ethnic communities

During 2023, the Race Equality Foundation held online discussions about end-of-life care for people from Black, Asian and minority ethnic backgrounds with a broad set of stakeholders from the public and health and social care. The aim was to identify pathways to improvement. Points of consensus were the need to:

- build trust between minority ethnic communities and healthcare providers
- prioritize person-centred care planning, including consideration of each person's cultural background, values and life history
- empower older immigrants by providing education on end-of-life care.

The report of one meeting (Butt & Race Equality Foundation, 2023) highlighted good practice examples that show ways to start conversations about advance care planning. The examples tend to use innovative methods, for example via art or humour, to allow people to break taboos around discussing death and enable people to approach advance care planning. One of the examples is described in the box below.

NO BARRIERS HERE©: AN ARTS-BASED APPROACH TO STARTING CONVERSATIONS ABOUT END-OF-LIFE CARE PLANNING

No Barriers Here is a small specialist organization with a team of people experienced in palliative care, arts-based psychotherapies and community engagement, which works alongside communities who experience inequalities (www.nobarriershere.org). In 2019, they worked with people living with learning disabilities to co-produce a series of three workshops to improve advance care planning and access to palliative and end-of-life care. The workshops have also been run with people from diverse ethnic backgrounds

(Jerwood & Allen, 2023), although there is no report of working with people living with dementia to date.

The three advance care planning workshops address the following:

- Who am I and what is important to me?
- Who are the important people in my life who can help me make decisions about my care?
- Where would I like to be cared for?
- What are the most important things about my future care?
- What are my funeral plans?
- What would I like my legacy to be?
- What has been important in my life?
- How would I like to be remembered?

The essence of the approach is to create safe spaces to have conversations about advance care planning through the use of arts-based activities that allow expression of views without form-filling.

> **POINT FOR PRACTICE: USE CREATIVE APPROACHES TO ENABLE CONVERSATIONS ABOUT FUTURE CARE**
>
> Talk with people from minority ethnic backgrounds who are living with dementia about their wishes for future care, earlier rather than later. If you are worried about how to do this, discuss it with someone from a palliative care team. Consider using indirect and creative approaches to enable people to think about and express their wishes.

End-of-life care
Palliative and end-of-life care for people with dementia
UK NHS ambitions for palliative and end-of-life care are laid out

in a national framework document (NHS England, 2022). The overarching ambition is phrased as an 'I' statement: 'I can make the last stage of my life as good as possible because everyone works together confidently, honestly and consistently to help me and the people who are important to me, including my carer(s)' (p.9).

Six aims are put forward to achieve this goal, including that each person is seen as an individual and gets fair access to care. However, at present, people with dementia are probably not getting equitable access. Only 20% of referrals for palliative and end-of-life care are for people with non-cancer diagnoses, including dementia. This may be partly due to the difficulty of knowing when a person with dementia is approaching death. A Social Care Institute for Excellence (SCIE) report (Manthorpe *et al.*, 2010) highlights repeated infections and rapid decline over hours or perhaps two or three weeks as signalling that a person with dementia is approaching end of life. The report recommends that if these signals are present, a doctor or nurse should be consulted so that an end-of-life plan can be formulated and put in place. However, dementia services in the UK are provided by mental health services, whereas palliative and end-of-life services are usually within acute NHS Trusts or hospice services. This means there can be a 'service gap' and lack of a clear care pathway between these services (Birch & Draper, 2008). The National Framework document, *Ambitions for palliative and end of life care: A national framework for local action 2021–2026* (National Palliative and End of Life Care Partnership, 2021), acknowledges these 'unacceptable inequities and inequalities' (p.42) and gives a call to action, saying, 'There is a collective responsibility on all of those involved in the commissioning and provision of end-of-life care to put this right' (p. 21).

Palliative and end-of-life care for minority ethnic people with dementia

A Better Health Briefing from the Race Equality Foundation on end-of-life care for people from minority ethnic populations with dementia gives an excellent overview of the current position, including a summary of current inequalities along with possible explanations (Koffman, 2018). In relation to palliative and end-of-life care generally (not specifically for dementia), there is some evidence of both poorer *access* to palliative care and poorer *quality* of care (Calanzani, Koffman & Higginson, 2013; Dixon *et al.*, 2015).

POORER ACCESS

Dixon *et al.* (2015) reviewed equity issues in palliative care and found evidence suggesting that older people from minority ethnic groups were less likely than the majority to receive specialist palliative care, though the gap appears quite narrow. They found that 4% of those receiving palliative care in England and Wales were from minority ethnic backgrounds, whereas Black and South Asian populations constitute 5.2% of over-65s in England and Wales (Office for National Statistics, 2023). Calanzani *et al.*'s comprehensive report, *Palliative and end of life care for Black, Asian and Minority Ethnic groups in the UK* (2013), collated findings of 45 reviews. They also concluded that people from minority ethnic populations have lower access to palliative and end-of-life care compared to White British people, as a result of:

- people from minority ethnic communities lacking knowledge of services
- information about services not being provided in relevant languages or formats
- people having previous experiences of poor care so being unwilling to access palliative and end-of-life care
- family and religious values clashing with the idea of hospice care
- lack of referrals by professionals to palliative and end-of-life services.

LOWER QUALITY

Dixon *et al.* and Calanzani *et al.* also both concluded that minority ethnic populations receive poorer end-of-life care than the White British (Marie Curie, 2014). Studies included in their reviews highlighted reports of:

- poor communication
- patients and families not being included in critical decisions

- poor management of symptoms, including pain.

Sampson *et al.* (2006) found people with dementia from minority ethnicities were prescribed fewer medications to alleviate their symptoms.

REASONS FOR POOR EXPERIENCES

A review over ten years ago found little research on the reasons for poorer experience, and few further relevant studies have been published since 2012 (Evans *et al.*, 2012). The reasons are likely to parallel those underlying inequities at other points of life with dementia, relating to the following:

- being an immigrant – meaning more likelihood of having limited understanding of English and less familiarity with care systems and entitlements
- experiencing prejudice – meaning less trust in services
- being in a care system that tends to cater for the majority – including assumptions about autonomy, open communication and confidentiality, and daily routines that may not accommodate preferences/routines of those from other cultures
- having different cultural values from the majority population – affecting acceptability of certain aspects of care, such as those related to whether men or women should deliver intimate care and those related to the involvement of extended family
- having different faith and religious beliefs – meaning certain aspects of care such as those related to prayer and end-of-life rituals are important but may be hard to implement.

In contrast to the UK, there have been many studies in the US comparing 'Black' and 'White' care preferences at end of life of 'patients' and family carers, though not for dementia specifically. These find that African-Americans tend to have a greater preference for continuing intervention even when death is approaching, compared to White Americans (e.g. (Phipps *et al.*, 2003; Johnson, 2013; Griggs, 2020). One American study found that continuing 'aggressive' interventions at end of life was associated with poorer quality of life for the dying person and poorer adjustment to bereavement in those left behind (Wright et al., 2008).

There is very limited information about whether people from minority ethnic groups in the UK have different care preferences from the majority population (Calanzani, Koffman & Higginson, et al., 2013; Dixon et al., 2015). Additionally, preferences held by people from minority ethnicities are likely to change across generations. One UK study which involved interviewing healthcare professionals about barriers and facilitators to end-of-life care planning in ethnic minority groups found that people of minority ethnicities had misconceptions about CPR which led them to feel it would not be a good idea to allow an order not to attempt resuscitation (Islam, Taylor & Faull, 2021).

Improving minority ethnic communities' experiences of palliative and end-of-life care
SERVICE SUPPORT

Despite the evidence of inequalities, it has been found that people from minority ethnic communities received support from a wide range of community services at end of life, including hospice at home, social workers, Marie Curie nurses and rapid response services (Dixon et al., 2015). They were more likely than their White counterparts to have home help, meals-on-wheels, community nursing and spiritual or emotional support. Minority ethnic people interviewed for a SCIE report (Manthorpe et al., 2010) voiced positive responses to receiving end-of-life care, including:

- 'Yes [nurses] have the hat of a professional but at that time, they are like a family member, like a friend.'
- 'It's just like having an extra pair of hands to help you, but it's a solid pair of hands and that's the difference.'
- 'Personally I can't understand why someone wouldn't want to have help when there's help available.'

A useful leaflet on addressing inequalities in end-of-life care for ethnic minorities has been produced by the Care Quality Commission (CQC, 2016).

> **POINT FOR PRACTICE: ENSURE PEOPLE ARE WELL INFORMED ABOUT END-OF-LIFE CARE**
>
> The information above highlights that many minority ethnic families are prepared to receive support from community services for a relative at end of life. It also shows the importance of raising health literacy through giving people accurate, understandable information about health procedures, so that they can make informed choices. It is important to talk through the range of services and interventions available, explain what each provides and consider with them whether they are culturally suitable or whether any particular adaptations need to be made. This includes ensuring that people are well informed about the consequences of seeking 'aggressive' treatments at end of life, since this may result in distress for both the person and the family.

GENERAL FRAMEWORKS AND GUIDANCE

Two broad sets of recommendations were put forward for service improvements in 2014 and are still relevant today. In *Next steps: Improving end of life care for Black, Asian and Minority Ethnic people in the UK*, the Marie Curie Foundation called for politicians, government bodies, policy-makers, commissioners and research funders to pay attention to the needs of minority ethnic communities by profiling needs, gathering relevant data, consultation and involvement, and demonstrating accountability (Marie Curie, 2014). They suggested a number of tools/strategies to make a difference, including:

- equality impact assessments of current and future service models
- better training in cultural competency for staff
- dissemination of best practice examples
- production of tailored information for minority ethnic communities.

One chance to get it right (Leadership Alliance for the Care of Dying People, 2014) focused specifically on dying. This report is not specific to dementia or minority ethnic communities but dementia and ethnicity could be considered in relation to each of five priorities:

- *Recognize* that the person is approaching death and make sure their needs and wishes are taken into account.
- *Communicate* sensitively with the person and significant others.
- *Involve* the person and significant others in treatment and care decisions in line with the person's wishes or best interests.
- *Support* families and others identified as important to understand and meet their needs as far as possible.
- *Plan* and compassionately enact a care plan that considers food and drink, control of symptoms, and spiritual, social and psychological support.

CLINICAL PRACTICE

A pre-existing framework can be used to guide a culturally sensitive assessment to inform end-of-life care. In a single case study, Mountford and Dening (2019) used the culturagram assessment framework (Goodorally, 2015) to understand an Italian 85-year-old and their family's views around end-of-life care and to enable development of a focused care plan (Mountford & Dening, 2019). The framework suggests exploring ten domains (see Table 7.1).

Table 7.1: Domains of the culturagram assessment framework (Goodorally, 2015)

Domains	
Time the person has lived in the community, including whether they feel settled	Communication abilities/issues
Reasons for moving to current location	Work and education (e.g., if young onset dementia, how important is it to keep working?)

cont.

Person's experiences of how services, care and communities responded to their help-seeking	Religious and spiritual needs
Health beliefs (e.g., regarding control, cure and coping with dementia)	Crisis events (e.g., any need to get back to country of origin regularly/urgently?)
Family functioning/dynamics (e.g., who makes decisions, who is in charge?)	Entitlements (does the person have all entitlements, have they done any advance planning?)

PREFERRED PLACE OF DEATH

A major issue in end-of-life care planning is to establish where the person wishes to die.

It has been found that those from minority ethnic groups in the UK are more likely than the majority population to die in hospital than in a care home but there were no differences in relation to the odds of dying in hospital rather than at home (Dixon *et al.*, 2015). These findings reflect preferences of people from minority ethnic communities for avoiding care homes and imply that admissions to hospital may be equitable across the population.

FAITH, RELIGION AND SPIRITUALITY

A comprehensive report was produced by Public Health England (2016), titled *Faith at end of life: A resource for professionals, providers and commissioners working in communities*. It aims to give enough understanding of the six major religions in England (Buddhism, Christianity, Hinduism, Islam, Judaism, Sikhism) for health and social care staff to be able to support holistic, person-centred, end-of-life care that takes faith into account. For each faith, it gives a very brief background and then focuses on practices and needs around the time of death and after death.

To give an example, the section on Hinduism briefly covers beliefs about how the cycle of birth, death and rebirth is influenced by karma. It describes Hindu rituals and beliefs as death approaches, including an emphasis on the state of mind of the dying person to help them in their subsequent rebirth and the provision of a final sacrament. The importance of state of mind may mean that the person wants certain religious objects around them or might benefit from the atmosphere created by chanting. It may also be important for extended family members to see the person before they die to ask forgiveness for any past misdeeds. Treatment of the body after death is also addressed, including timing of cremation, characteristics of the mourning period and dispersal of the ashes. The text also explains that Hinduism designates certain days as 'sraddha' days, which are for remembering ancestors, raising money for charity and giving offerings to priests to help the soul on its journey.

Understanding the basics of the religious faith of a family when someone is dying in a hospital or care home setting can help you to make appropriate arrangements that enable the person to have 'a good death'. For example, this might include:

- planning the layout of the room to accommodate items needed and ensuring that the person is facing the right way
- contacting an appropriate religious figure to administer sacraments at the right time
- making arrangements to cater for expected numbers of visitors
- planning for the time immediately after death and involving family where possible in cultural practices around laying out of the body.

As in other areas of practice, it is important to be attuned to the individual to make sure you don't make stereotypical assumptions. This was articulately expressed by a GP in one study, who said:

> So, you have to be careful that you don't say, 'Somebody is a Sikh, therefore, they will react in this way.' What you have to say is they have a belief system, but they will have a variable belief system.
> *(Islam, Taylor & Faull, 2021, p.e622)*

Public Health England provides a useful set of recommendations to follow when formulating end-of-life care plans. The recommendations are shown in Table 7.2.

Table 7.2: Key recommendations for health and care professionals formulating end-of-life care plans for people from minority ethnic communities

Ensure that information and services are provided in the preferred language for the person and their family.
Establish the best words for talking with the person and family about plans, considering whether to use direct terms like death and dying or not.
Find out about the role of family members in putting together the care plan.
Identify whether the person or family has religious beliefs or spiritual needs that they wish to be taken into account and make a record of these.
Find out whether the person and/or their family would like access to religious or spiritual support and, if so, who from.
Access support from colleagues, religious leaders or chaplains on issues you are uncertain about.

Adapted from Faith at end of life: A resource for professionals, providers and commissioners working in communities (Public Health England, 2016).

> **POINT FOR PRACTICE: CO-DEVELOP ETHNICALLY APPROPRIATE CARE PLANS**
> Palliative and end-of-life care experiences of minority ethnic populations are poorer than for the majority population, but we cannot identify isolated reasons for this. Therefore, this highlights the importance of:
>
> - paying special attention to palliative and end-of-life care planning with people with dementia and their families from these communities
> - co-developing, through discussion with the person (where possible) and their family, an individual person-centred care plan that takes all aspects of ethnicity into account.

Being bereaved of a relative with dementia

In this section, we look at the context of being bereaved of a relative with dementia, consider how culture and religion affect grieving, and explore the role of health and care professionals in helping people of minority ethnicities to adapt.

The death of a person with dementia is a major turning point for families. A lot of research has looked at the human response to bereavement, leading to evidence-supported theories about how we come to terms with loss. These have moved beyond the idea that people get over a loss stage-by-stage over time. Rather, grieving has been found to involve pendulum swings between confronting loss (which puts the person in touch with feelings of grief) and blocking loss (which enables the person to get on with life) (Stroebe & Schut, 1999). It is widely accepted that feelings of grief can be re-triggered by particular dates, events or experiences across many years. The majority of people access support from their own resources and friends and family to help them adapt. However, about one in five struggle to come to terms and may benefit from specialist support.

Pre-death factors affecting caregiver grief

Three pre-death factors are particularly relevant to families who are bereaved of someone with dementia: chronic sorrow, anticipatory grief and consequences of caregiving.

CHRONIC SORROW

Witnessing progressive loss can cause 'chronic sorrow', often over many years; for example, a carer may feel grief when the person has to give up driving, grief in response to the person not recognizing a grandchild, grief in response to them needing help with dressing and so on. Expressing this sorrow to someone who can understand seems to lessen its burden (Hoppe, 2018). However, in minority ethnic communities where stigma is high, those who are providing care may hide their sorrow, for fear of appearing as if they are struggling to fulfil the expected duty of caring. Also, lack of knowledge about dementia may result in lack of sympathy for carers from extended family members (Rauf, 2023). This means many minority ethnic carers may not be offered empathic support and may carry the burden of their sorrow within themselves. Someone in this position may feel isolated and exhausted by the point of bereavement.

ANTICIPATORY GRIEF

'Anticipatory grief' refers to grieving a death before it has happened (Fulton & Gottesman, 1980). This is not uncommon because, in advanced dementia, relatives often feel as if they have already lost the person, so they grieve even though the person is still alive. This is experienced by about half to three-quarters of carers (Chan *et al.*, 2013). Anticipatory grief implies that the emotional bonds between the person living with dementia and family members are already loosening prior to death. This may or may not be good for the relationship. On one hand, some emotional detachment may enable carers to continue to care without becoming distraught. On the other hand, if the person with dementia is depersonalized, this can lead to un-empathic care (Riley, Evans & Oyebode, 2018). Research suggests anticipatory grieving leads to a less intense grief reaction at the point of death.

One research study in the US showed that the African-American population had lower levels of anticipatory grief than the White population and were more vulnerable to stronger grief at the point of death (Owen, Goode & Haley, 2001; Chan *et al.*, 2013). Considering the minority ethnic communities in the UK, it seems possible that there would be less anticipatory grief because the individual with dementia more often stays with the family than in a care home. We know that the move to a care home is a point at which many adult-child carers experience anticipatory grief and some emotional detachment (Ott, Sanders & Kelber, 2007).

CONSEQUENCES OF CAREGIVING

Caring for someone with advanced dementia may become all-consuming. This can lead to a crisis of identity when a former carer no longer has a caring role. Our studies in the South Asian community in Bradford suggest that in many families care is shared between siblings, enabling them to continue other roles, for example as spouse, mother and employee (Parveen, Blakey & Oyebode, 2018; Rauf, 2023). Perhaps where there is shared family caregiving, it may be that family members have less of an identity crisis when the person with dementia dies than where the care predominantly falls on one individual.

> **POINT FOR PRACTICE: OFFER A FOLLOW-UP APPOINTMENT AFTER BEREAVEMENT**
> After the death of a person with dementia, health and social care workers who have been involved usually end contact with the person's family. However, if there is opportunity for a follow-up appointment, it is worth using this to gauge whether those who are bereaved will struggle to adapt.

A key issue for people from minority ethnicities may be whether the carer expressed any chronic sorrow during the lifetime of the person with dementia. Those who have not been able to openly communicate this with other family members or friends may be more vulnerable to struggle after bereavement. It can be helpful to signpost anyone in this position to future sources of peer support, if they do not have family members or friends to confide in.

Post-death factors affecting adjustment to bereavement
RITUAL

In individualistic societies such as the UK, people nowadays have freedom to mourn as they wish without pressure to conform to one right way. In more traditional societies, referred to as 'collectivist', those who are bereaved are expected to follow certain customs to ensure the harmony of the group, in terms of the timing and type of funeral, the mourning period and the expression of grief.

Many first-generation migrants have come to the UK from collectivist societies and many have retained these values in the UK. Members of these communities may find performing rituals provides a helpful structure in the period after bereavement but some may find others' expectations stifling or wish they had quiet time to themselves and space to grieve in their own way. It also needs to be remembered that in our super-diverse society, some migrants may neither feel part of the majority British society, nor have an established ethnic community to relate to. These people, in particular, are likely to be vulnerable after a bereavement.

RELIGION

Religious faith is central to the lives of many people from minority ethnicities. Religion has a major influence on rituals concerning death and mourning and on beliefs about whether the deceased is at peace. Religious faith can also give feelings of comfort and solace. A review of dementia caregivers' grief noted that those with religious beliefs were less likely to have a complicated grief reaction and were more likely to feel prepared for the death of their relative (Chan *et al.*, 2013).

CONTINUING BONDS

Cultural and religious beliefs influence whether bereaved families have a 'continuing bond' with the deceased (Klass, Silverman & Nickman, 2014). In the UK and many western societies, there has been an expectation that people 'get over' a death and sever bonds with the deceased. However, in other societies, it is accepted that emotional bonds are retained with those who have died. These bonds may be:

- personal, for example the living still talk to/with the deceased
- social, for example family members readily talk together about the person who died
- spiritual, for example looking after the well-being of the person who has died through prayer, giving or other offerings or through holding the belief that ancestors are still present in the lives of the living.

> **POINT FOR PRACTICE: ASK ABOUT MOURNING RITUALS**
>
> In considering whether bereaved carers or families need support to adapt to life without the person, health and care professionals may find it useful to:

- ask about cultural and religious beliefs and practices
- establish whether the person is able to follow those rituals if they wish to
- explore whether they lack support or find their cultural obligations stressful or burdensome.

You could signpost to religious advisors or psychosocial interventions/support as indicated.

Conclusion

In this chapter, we have looked at special considerations around care for those with dementia and their families from minority ethnicities in relation to advance care planning, end-of-life care and bereavement.

Advance care planning involves talking about, and possibly writing down, the way you would like to be cared for towards the end of life. It can include advance directives to refuse certain treatments as well as statements about preferences for places or types of care that would and would not be acceptable. Little is known about advance care planning in relation to minority ethnicities but a number of issues may be barriers to its use. The barriers may relate to cultural and religious beliefs, lack of awareness of how dementia develops, lack of knowledge of legal frameworks, lack of trust in services, and staff lacking the knowledge, competencies and confidence to address the area. However, there are some examples of how advance care planning can be approached for minority ethnic communities, and use of creative approaches is prominent in these.

In relation to palliative and end-of-life care, people from minority ethnic communities who are dying from dementia probably do not get equitable access to this type of care, and there are reports of poor-quality care. Multiple factors may contribute to inequities, so it is important that health and care staff take proactive steps to talk about and co-develop timely person-centred and family-centred end-of-life care plans. There are some suggested signals that can prompt addressing end-of-life care in a timely way. Despite the lack of specific research, there are broad frameworks and some guidance to inform how to provide good-quality end-of-life care for those from minority ethic communities. Particular issues include establishing the preferred place of death and identifying cultural and religious practices around dying that need to be accommodated within end-of-life care.

Following bereavement, most people access support from their own resources, friends and family to help them adapt, but about 20% struggle and may benefit from specialist support.

There is little known about pre-bereavement influences on adjustment in minority ethnic carers or families following the death of someone with dementia. It is possible that anticipatory grief is lower (because it is less likely the person will move into care) and that chronic sorrow is not expressed due to stigma. These factors could increase the intensity of grief following bereavement. There is equally little research regarding post-bereavement influences on adjustment. Cultural rituals, religion and continuing bonds with the deceased may be helpful, but generalized assumptions cannot be made. Rather than immediately discharging from support services when the 'index person' dies, it can be helpful to follow up and signpost those who may be vulnerable to appropriate sources of support.

Chapter 8

Conclusions

In this book, we have summarized what is known about how being from a minority ethnic group in the UK influences the risk of developing dementia, perceptions of dementia, experiences of assessment and diagnosis, and life with the condition. We have interwoven the implications for health and social care staff who provide dementia care services and support. In this final brief chapter, we summarize the key points arising.

Following the introduction in Chapter 1, Chapters 2 and 3 stressed the importance of those in minority ethnic communities being aware of dementia. In Chapter 2, this was in relation to awareness of avoidable risk factors. In Chapter 3, it was in relation to knowledge and awareness of the nature of dementia itself. In both these areas, we saw that it would benefit minority ethnic communities to develop further awareness. Lack of awareness and misunderstandings about the causes of dementia create stigma and shame, and lead to delays in seeking help.

In the following four chapters, we focused on the trajectory of dementia, from assessment and diagnosis, to living with dementia in the community, to living with dementia in a care home, and finally to the end of life and bereavement of a family member with dementia. In all these areas, research has identified that families from minority ethnic communities face barriers to accessing services. These barriers are at individual level, community level and service level. They prevent or make it harder for people from minority ethnic backgrounds to get the support they need.

To address the health inequities in relation to dementia care in minority ethnic communities, it is vitally important to address the barriers that are experienced both at an individual level (including lack of awareness) and as a result of barriers to accessing services (service level). Below, we summarize key points emerging from our review of evidence and accounts of experience from people of minority ethnicities, across the journey with dementia.

There is increasing emphasis from researchers and policy-makers on the links between dementia and lifestyle, with the hope that changing aspects of lifestyle may reduce the risk of developing dementia. We addressed this area in Chapter 2. We noted that minority ethnic communities have increased risk in relation to seven of the 14 modifiable risk factors that have been identified. These are that they have a higher prevalence of diabetes, hypertension, obesity and depression, are less likely to engage in physical activity, and are more likely to experience loneliness. These statistics are based on population comparisons and do not mean each individual of minority ethnicity lives a lifestyle that carries these risks. It also does not mean everyone could avoid developing dementia by avoiding all the modifiable risks. However, it does provide an incentive to consider how individuals and communities can be encouraged to reduce risks.

We introduced the Theoretical Domains Framework as a useful way of thinking about how to help communities or individuals make changes in lifestyle to reduce risk. Its four key steps are: to identify the most impactful behaviour to change, to identify the barriers to making changes, to select a behaviour change technique that is matched with the particular barriers, and to evaluate what happens and adjust as needed. Although there is no evidence to date that community-level mass media campaigns are effective in reducing dementia risk in minority ethnic communities, there are some ways to try and ensure that campaigns directed at behaviour change in these communities have the best chance of being effective. In particular, it is important to clearly identify the specific minority ethnic audience, to deliver simple key messages through targeted channels appropriate to that audience, and to include a clear call to action. On an individual level, the most effective and cheapest interventions to reduce the risk of dementia are nicotine replacement therapy, anti-hypertension medication and provision of hearing aids. Raising community and individual awareness of the importance of healthy lifestyles throughout the life course is an important step towards reducing health inequalities.

If and when dementia develops, awareness and understanding of dementia itself is vital to reduce the stigma and encourage people to seek help and support. We considered awareness and understanding of dementia within minority ethnic communities in Chapter 3. Perceptions of dementia within minority ethnic communities in the UK may be changing, with some evidence of increased awareness that dementia is a disease of the brain often associated with memory problems. However, the causes of dementia and the nature of advanced symptoms are often still misunderstood. The condition may be thought of as normal ageing, a punishment from God or as being caused by jinns or spirits. Symptoms of advanced dementia, including confused speech or hallucinations, may be misidentified as 'madness', which in many minority ethnic communities carries high levels of stigma. This can lead to people hiding their symptoms, families isolating the individual from social contact for fear of embarrassment, and the person and family not seeking a diagnosis, so being unable to access treatment or support. Ultimately, this may lead to many people from minority ethnic communities with dementia having a poorer quality of life compared to the majority population.

Understanding specific misconceptions related to dementia in minority ethnic communities is key to designing culturally sensitive and effective dementia awareness programmes. When adapting dementia awareness materials for a specific cultural group there needs to be consideration of the *content* of the information, ensuring that it uses culturally meaningful words, examples and images. In many languages there is no word for dementia, so dementia has often been translated as 'memory problems'. This has been found to cause misunderstanding, given that dementia affects much more then memory, so is to be avoided. A format needs to be chosen via which awareness-raising content will be presented. Although research has focused on leaflets, they have limited value for minority ethnic communities. There is instead a preference for face-to-face education in a community setting from bilingual community workers, or professionally qualified staff with language abilities. Once there is content and a medium for delivery, a decision also needs to be made about a suitable setting – this could be a neutral accessible place, such as a community centre, a place of worship or attending a community event or meeting. In all these aspects, it is important to work jointly with communities to co-produce relevant, culturally meaningful campaigns.

There is some evidence that people of minority ethnicities have poorer cognitive functioning at the point of a diagnosis of dementia. This may be partly because, due to lack of awareness and lack of trust in a helpful response, people approach services later than those from a White British background. However, once a person affected, or their family member, seeks help for possible dementia from a GP, processes of assessment and diagnosis should then take place. This area is covered in Chapter 4 where we saw that there are community-related and service-related barriers that prevent equitable access to dementia assessment services but that there are also ways to overcome these. Targeted communication about dementia and dementia assessment to older people from their own GP has been shown to encourage people to approach services for assessment. Offering appointments with professionals who speak community languages may also reduce reluctance to come forward. It may be helpful too for primary care staff, such as practice nurses, who are seeing someone about other physical health problems, such as diabetes, to take a proactive role by being vigilant to cognitive issues, so they can raise the benefits of assessment if appropriate.

We also noted in Chapter 4 that there are many reasons why older people from minority ethnic backgrounds may hesitate to give an open account of their difficulties, so it is vital to take time to build a trusting relationship before conducting a formal assessment. If a person attending a dementia assessment service does not speak English and there isn't a bilingual professional available, communicating via a professional interpreter may be preferable to going through a family member.

The attitudes and behaviours of professionals and the tools they have to help with accurate diagnosis can all be service-related barriers to assessment. Rates of referral from GPs to dementia assessment services vary, with people of some minority ethnicities not being referred in the numbers expected, perhaps partly due to staff fears of causing upset or assuming that diagnosis would be unwelcome. Compared with the White British population, it appears that rates of diagnosis are lower in people from South Asian communities and higher in Black populations. One contributing issue is that cognitive screening tests are not valid across all cultural groups and may produce false positives, implying acquired cognitive difficulties where there are none. We noted that the ACE, MoCA and RUDAS are the recommended cognitive assessment tools for use with people from minority ethnic communities. However, scores should always be used with caution. We also noted that it is important to use culturally and personally meaningful tasks when assessing functional abilities. Family structures and gender roles may be different in ethnic minority communities from those in the majority community, so it is important when gathering information from family members to be aware of extended family dynamics and seek to talk with those who provide the hands-on care as well the family spokesperson.

In Chapter 5, we moved on to consider the influences of ethnicity on care in the community. It is difficult to establish the number of family carers from minority ethnic communities, as caregiving is seen as an expected family responsibility and not a special role, so the label 'carer' may not be used. We looked at the evidence that cultural values, such as familism which tends to be strong in many minority ethnic communities, influence whether a person adopts the carer role, how the person perceives that role and how they cope with it. In many minority ethnic communities, families feel culturally obliged to provide care. However, feeling obliged to care does not mean families are also willing and prepared for what this involves. Where family carers are obliged yet reluctant or unprepared, this may lead to a poorer quality of life for the carer and also for the person with dementia. We noted that culturally sensitive post-diagnostic support services are both desired and required to help minority ethnic carers be prepared and manage over time.

As with barriers to assessment and diagnosis, minority ethnic families also face barriers to accessing post-diagnostic support. Drawing on research, we put forward key recommendations for reducing these barriers. We stressed the importance of working in partnership with communities and across service sectors, culturally adapting existing services and interventions, actively promoting services, managing language aspects and upskilling the workforce. Having culturally competent staff is key for providing person-centred care and promoting trust and collaboration between families and health and social care professionals.

Preparation for taking on caring can help carers have a more positive experience. People from minority ethnicities believe it is possible to 'live well' with dementia but stress their wish to have information and support to help them with a wide range of aspects of care. Some specific psychosocial interventions, such as cognitive stimulation, reminiscence and carer information programmes, have been adapted to make them suitable for particular ethnicities. However, there is a need for further work to extend the number of adapted interventions and evaluate their acceptability and benefits.

While there may be a grain of truth in the idea that people from minority ethnic communities 'look after their own', this is not always practically possible due to changing family networks caused by shifts in immigration policies and the economic necessities of going out to work. Changes in families, as second- and third-generation immigrants adapt to UK societal influences, may mean family care is becoming less available. In Chapter 6 of the book, we consider the issue of minority ethnicities and care homes. Although people from ethnic minorities tend not to be positive about using care homes, a significant number of people with advanced dementia from minority ethnic backgrounds do move into care due to issues of safeguarding or heavy care needs. These decisions can be hard to make. Different family members may have different views, and different amounts of power to make their views known. Therefore, staff need to find ways of enabling families to talk openly together about the issues to reach a consensus. Stigma is still commonly faced by families who place a relative in a care home. Services need to support families who face isolation or stigma from their own community when a relative moves into a care home. We noted that families may appreciate being in touch with others in a similar situation.

With few culture-specific care homes, there are challenges to accessing culturally appropriate care. In order to support individuals and families from minority ethnic communities well, staff in health and social care roles need to be aware of their own assumptions or generalizations, for example that all South Asian care home residents love hot spicy food. Key issues for care home staff are finding out about the needs, likes and dislikes of minority ethnic residents with regard to communication, social connections and activities, food and faith. It can be very isolating for someone from a minority ethnic background to be in a care home, where they may share little in terms of personal experiences with other residents. To combat this, it is essential to find ways to communicate, especially with those who do not speak English or who lose their English language. One way to help staff feel confident to meet the needs of residents from minority ethnic backgrounds is to promote collaborations between care homes and minority ethnic organizations, who can provide helpful information and assist with communication. In addition, all staff need to be able to challenge racism if staff or residents in a care home express prejudice. Research on how best to meet the needs of people from minority ethnicities in care homes is under-developed and more is needed, but overall, it supports the notion that staff training and collaboration with organizations from minority ethnic communities are the keys to culturally sensitive care.

Dementia is a life-shortening condition. Although many people with dementia, especially those from minority ethnic backgrounds, live with multi-morbidities (i.e., with other conditions as well as dementia), many die as a result of the impact of dementia on their health. In Chapter 7 of the book, we addressed issues around the end of life. Paradoxically, research shows that people with dementia from a wide range of minority ethnicities, including White Irish, survive longer with dementia than the majority population, although it is possible that this effect is linked with the good health of first-generation migrants. This is important to note, as it means minority ethnic families support relatives with dementia over a longer period than the White British and therefore advance care planning may be especially relevant.

There is very little research on ethnicity and advance care

planning but we surmised that there could be a number of special considerations, including that delay to diagnosis means those with dementia have a narrower window of time in which they can make their own decisions while having mental capacity to do so. In addition, cultural and religious beliefs, lack of knowledge of UK legal systems and lack of trust in healthcare may all be barriers to making advance care plans. We noted that recent consultations with people of minority ethnic communities attempted to overcome these by building trusting relationships, providing information on the end of life, and prioritising person-centred care planning.

There is evidence that people from minority ethnic backgrounds have poorer access to palliative care and poorer quality of care, including poorer management of symptoms and lack of communication with the person and family members. On the other hand, research shows people from ethnic minorities do receive and appreciate a wide range of community palliative care services. To improve end-of-life care for minority ethnic families, it is important to offer accurate information about palliative care services and interventions, consult about whether any particular cultural adaptations to care need to be made, and find out whether there are religious rituals that would enable the person to have a 'good death'.

There are also some special considerations concerning support for families bereaved of someone with dementia. People from minority ethnic communities may not express sorrow during the person's lifetime as this may be culturally unacceptable, and they may also experience less anticipatory grief than White British people, not least as they may not be separated if the person with dementia does not move into care. In this sense, people from minority ethnicities may experience sudden grief when the person dies. On the other hand, if care has been shared between siblings, as would be the case in many minority ethnic families, it is possible family carers would not experience the loss of identity that is felt when care has been carried by one person. Religion is important in the process of grieving for those with faith, so it is vital to ensure that care systems support necessary rituals. It may also be helpful for care professionals to provide a listening ear for those who find this aspect difficult.

In addition to considering the common issue of barriers to care that we emphasized at the start of this chapter, we need further research on a number of topics connected with minority ethnicities and dementia care, including the development and evaluation of culturally adapted interventions and services. We need a well-trained workforce, which is aware of bias and confident to enquire about cultural issues, if we are to be able to deliver culturally acceptable care. Finally, we must acknowledge the importance of developing trusting relationships whether at individual or community level. Open communication and co-production are vital to overcoming barriers and making meaningful adaptations to services.

In this book, in addition to summarizing published research, we have drawn on our own studies and on the words of those who have given their time to help us understand the experiences and needs of minority ethnic communities in the UK. We hope members of communities who read the book find information that is relevant, and that health and care professionals can use the material to enhance their own culturally competent care.

Appendix: Matching Behaviour Change Techniques to Barriers (Michie *et al.*, 2011)

Barriers	Behaviour change technique (BCT) label and definition	Example of applying the BCT in dementia care
Knowledge Beliefs about consequences Motivation and goals	**BCT 1. Provide general information on behaviour–health link** Information about the relationship between the behaviour and health OR health education material relevant to the behaviour.	Provide information about the link between type 2 diabetes and dementia, showing how risk of dementia increases if diabetes is not well controlled.
Knowledge Beliefs about consequences Motivation and goals	**BCT 2. Provide information on consequences** Provide information focusing on what will happen if the person changes or does not change their behaviour.	Provide information about how lack of physical activity can lead to obesity and vascular dementia but being active can reduce weight and so reduce risk.

Social and professional role and identity Beliefs about capabilities Motivation and goals Social influences	**BCT 3. Provide information about others' approval** Provide information about what other people think about the target person's behaviour and whether others will approve or disapprove of what the person is doing or will do.	Use posters of well-known community leaders/influencers advocating the behaviour (e.g., encouraging going on a run in the park).
Skills Beliefs about capabilities Action planning	**BCT 4. Prompt intention formation** Encourage the person to set a general goal or make a behavioural resolution, expressed as a specific goal that involves action. This encourages people to decide to change.	Ask the person to write out a goal: 'I will walk for 30 minutes every day' or 'I will only eat cake at weekends.'

References

Action on Smoking and Health. (2024). Factsheet: *Tobacco and ethnic minorities*. Retrieved 11 October 2024 from: https://ash.org.uk/resources/view/tobacco-and-ethnic-minorities

Adelman, S. *et al.* (2011). Prevalence of dementia in African-Caribbean compared with UK-born White older people: Two-stage cross-sectional study. *British Journal of Psychiatry*, 199(2), 119–125.

Age UK. (n.d). Loneliness. www.ageuk.org.uk/information-advice/health-wellbeing/loneliness

Akarsu, N.E. *et al.* (2019). Depression in carers of people with dementia from a minority ethnic background: Systematic review and meta-analysis of randomised controlled trials of psychosocial interventions. *International Journal of Geriatric Psychiatry*, 34(6), 790–806.

All Party Parliamentary Group on Dementia. (2013). *Dementia does not discriminate: the experiences of black, Asian and minority ethnic communities*. London: The Stationery Office.

Alzheimer's Disease International. (2024). *World Alzheimer Report 2024: Global changes in attitudes to dementia*. London: Alzheimer's Disease International.

Alzheimer's Research UK. (2015). *Dementia in the family: The impact on carers*. Cambridge: ARUK. Retrieved 12 October 2024 from: www.alzheimersresearchuk.org/about-us/our-influence/policy-work/reports/carers-report

Alzheimer's Society. (2021). *This is me*. Third edition. Retrieved 15 October 2024 from: www.alzheimers.org.uk/get-support/publications-factsheets/this-is-me

Arblaster, K. (2021). *Ethnic minority communities: Increasing access to a dementia diagnosis*. Retrieved 12 October 2024 from: www.alzheimers.org.uk/sites/default/files/2021-09/ethinic_minorities_increasing_access_to_diagnosis.pdf

Aspinall, P.J. (2020). Ethnic/racial terminology as a form of representation: A critical review of the lexicon of collective and specific terms in use in Britain. *Genealogy*, 4(3), 87.

Badger, F. *et al.* (2012). A survey of issues of ethnicity and culture in nursing homes in an English region: Nurse managers' perspectives. *Journal of Clinical Nursing*, 21(11–12), 1726–1735.

Baillie, L., Beecraft, S. & Woods, S. (2015). Dementia Friends sessions for nursing students. *Nursing Older People*, 27(9), 34–38.

Banerjee, S. *et al.* (2003). Predictors of institutionalisation in people with dementia. *Journal of Neurology, Neurosurgery and Psychiatry*, 74(9), 1315–1316.

Berning, M.J. *et al.* (2023). Effect of a dementia friends information session on health professional students' attitudes and knowledge related to dementia. *Gerontology & Geriatrics Education*, 44, 185–195.

REFERENCES

Berwald, S. et al. (2016). Black African and Caribbean British communities' perceptions of memory problems: 'We don't do dementia'. *PLoS One*, 11(4), e0151878.

Bifarin, O.O. (2022). *Intersections between culture, sociodemographic change and caring: A qualitative study of current and prospective family caregivers in mainland China*. https://bradscholars.brad.ac.uk/entities/publication/b7a57d6f-8d14-44f7-a5cd-5627cab815ee

Birch, D. & Draper, J. (2008). A critical literature review exploring the challenges of delivering effective palliative care to older people with dementia. *Journal of Clinical Nursing*, 17(9), 1144–1163.

Blakemore, A. et al. (2018). Dementia in UK South Asians: A scoping review of the literature. *BMJ Open*, 8(4), e020290.

Blakey, H., Parveen, S. & Oyebode, J. (2016). Does size matter? The benefits and challenges of voluntary sector partnerships in dementia service provision for South Asian communities in England. *Voluntary Sector Review*, 7(2), 1891–208.

Bothongo, P.L. et al. (2022). Dementia risk in a diverse population: A single-region nested case-control study in the East End of London. *The Lancet Regional Health – Europe*, 15, 100321.

Brayne, C. et al. (2006). Medical Research Council Cognitive Function and Ageing Study Investigators. Dementia before death in ageing societies – the promise of prevention and the reality. *PLoS Medicine*, 3(10), e397.

Brodaty, H., Seeher, K. & Gibson, L. (2012). Dementia time to death: A systematic literature review on survival time and years of life lost in people with dementia. *International Psychogeriatrics*, (24)7, 1034–1045.

Brottman, M.R. et al. (2020). Toward cultural competency in health care: A scoping review of the diversity and inclusion education literature. *Academic Medicine*, 95(5), 803–813.

Buschke, H. et al. (1999). Screening for dementia with the memory impairment screen. *Neurology*, 52(2), 231–238.

Cahill, K.M. et al. (2021). Familism values and adjustment among Hispanic/Latino individuals: A systematic review and meta-analysis. *Psychological Bulletin*, 147(9), 947–985.

Calanzani, N., Koffman, J. & Higginson, I. (2013). *Palliative and end of life care for Black, Asian and Minority Ethnic groups in the UK: Demographic profile and the current state of palliative and end of life care provision*. London: Public Health England.

Capstick, A. et al. (2021). Drawn from life: Cocreating narrative and graphic vignettes of lived experience with people affected by dementia. *Health Expectations*, 24(5), 1890–1900.

Care Act (2014). Retrieved 12 October 2024 from: www.legislation.gov.uk/ukpga/2014/23/contents

Care Quality Commission (CQC). (2016). *People from Black and minority ethnic communities. A different ending: Addressing inequalities in end of life care*. Retrieved 20 October 2024 from: www.cqc.org.uk/sites/default/files/20160505%20CQC_EOLC_BAME_FINAL_2.pdf

Carers UK (2023). *Supporting Black, Asian and minority ethnic carers: A good practice briefing*. Retrieved 12 October 2024 from: www.carersuk.org/media/3izluvum/cuk-black-asian-and-minority-ethnic-carers-good-practice-briefing.pdf

Chan, D. et al. (2013). Grief reactions in dementia carers: A systematic review. *International Journal of Geriatric Psychiatry*, 28(1), 1–17.

Co, M. et al. (2021). Differences in survival and mortality in minority ethnic groups with dementia: A systematic review and meta-analysis. *International Journal of Geriatric Psychiatry*, 6(11), 640–1663.

Co, M. et al. (2023) Ethnicity and survival after a dementia diagnosis: A retrospective cohort study using electronic health record data. *Alzheimer's Research & Therapy*, 15(1), 67.

Collins, L. (2020). *Understanding the eating and drinking experiences of people living with dementia and dysphagia in care homes: A qualitative study of the multiple perspectives of the person, their family, care home staff and speech and language therapists*. Doctoral dissertation, University of Bradford.

Cook, L. et al. (2019). Parity of access to memory services in London for the BAME population: A cross-sectional study. *Aging & Mental Health*, 23(6), 693–697.

Cooper, C. et al. (2018). Relationship between speaking English as a second language and agitation in people with dementia living in care homes: Results from the MARQUE (Managing Agitation and Raising Quality of life) English national care home survey. *International Journal of Geriatric Psychiatry*, 33(3), 504–509.

Cordell, C.B. et al. (2013). Alzheimer's Association recommendations for operationalizing the detection of cognitive impairment during. *Alzheimer's & Dementia*, 9(2), 141–150.

Cova, I. et al. (2022). Translations and cultural adaptations of the Montreal Cognitive Assessment: A systematic and qualitative review. *Neurological Science*, 43(1), 113–124.

Cuibus, M.V. (2024). Migrants in the UK: An overview. Regional Ethnic Diversity. Gov.UK. Retrieved 4 October 2024 from: https://migrationobservatory.ox.ac.uk/wp-content/uploads/2017/02/MigObs-Briefing-Migrants-in-the-UK-an-overview-2024.pdf

Dahlgren, G. & Whitehead, M. (2021). The Dahlgren-Whitehead model of health determinants: 30 years on and still chasing rainbows. *Public Health*, 199, 20–24.

Dementia, UK. (2007). *A report to the Alzheimer's Society on the prevalence and economic cost of dementia in the UK*. King's College London and the London School of Economics.

Department of Health and Social Care. (2009). *Living Well With Dementia: A national dementia strategy*. www.gov.uk/government/publications/living-well-with-dementia-a-national-dementia-strategy

Department of Health and Social Care. (2012). *Prime Minister's challenge on dementia*. www.gov.uk/government/publications/prime-ministers-challenge-on-dementia

Department of Health and Social Care. (2015). *Prime Minister's Challenge on Dementia 2020*. www.gov.uk/government/publications/prime-ministers-challenge-on-dementia-2020

Devonport, T.J. et al. (2023). A systematic review of inequalities in the mental health experiences of Black African, Black Caribbean and Black-mixed UK populations: Implications for action. *Journal of Racial and Ethnic Health Disparities*, 10(4), 1669–1681.

Dixon, J. et al. (2015). *Equity in the provision of palliative care in the UK: Review of evidence*. Personal Social Services Research Unit and London School of Economics and Political Science.

Dlamini, T. (2021). *End of life care and dementia: A hermeneutic phenomenological exploration of community-dwelling Black African-Caribbean older people living with dementia and family carers*. Doctoral thesis, University of Huddersfield. Available from eprints.hud.ac.uk

REFERENCES

Evans, N. et al. (2012). Systematic review of the primary research on minority ethnic groups and end-of-life care from the United Kingdom. *Journal of Pain and Symptom Management*, 43(2), 261–286.

Fischer, A.G. (2001). *Assessment of Motor and Process Skills: Volume 1, Development, Standardization, and Administration*. Fort Collins, CO: Tree Star Press.

Folstein, M.F., Folstein, S.E. & McHugh, P.R. (1975). 'Mini-mental state.' A practical method for grading the cognitive state of patients for the clinician. *Journal of Psychiatric Research*, 12(3), 89–198.

Fulton, R. & Gottesman, D.J. (1980). Anticipatory grief: A psychosocial concept reconsidered. *British Journal of Psychiatry*, 137, 45–54.

Giebel, C.M. et al. (2019). Age, memory loss and perceptions of dementia in South Asian ethnic minorities. *Aging & Mental Health*, 23(2), 173–182.

Goodorally, V. (2015). Access, Assessment and Engagement. In J. Botsford & K. Harrison Dening (eds), *Dementia, Culture and Ethnicity: Issues for All*, (127–140). London: Jessica Kingsley Publishers.

Gove, D. et al. (2021). The challenges of achieving timely diagnosis and culturally appropriate care of people with dementia from minority ethnic groups in Europe. *International Journal of Geriatric Psychiatry*, 36(12), 1823–1828.

Griggs, J.J. (2020). Disparities in palliative care in patients with cancer. *Journal of Clinical Oncology*, 38(9), 974–979.

Hailstone, J. et al. (2017). The development of Attitudes of People from Ethnic Minorities to Help-Seeking for Dementia (APEND): A questionnaire to measure attitudes to help-seeking for dementia in people from South Asian backgrounds in the UK. *International Journal of Geriatric Psychiatry*, 32(3), 288–296.

Hodges, J.R. & Larner, A.J. (2017). Addenbrooke's Cognitive Examinations: ACE, ACE-R, ACE-III, ACEapp, and M-ACE. In A.J. Larner (ed.), *Cognitive Screening Instruments*. Cham: Springer.

Holt-Lunstad, J. (2020). Social isolation and health. *Health Affairs*. www.healthaffairs.org/do/10.1377/forefront.20200622.758097

Hoppe, S.A. (2018). Sorrow shared is a sorrow halved: The search for empathetic understanding of family members of a person with early-onset dementia. *Culture, Medicine, and Psychiatry*, 2(1), 180–201.

Hossain, M.Z. & Khan, H.T.A. (2020). Barriers to access and ways to improve dementia services for a minority ethnic group in England. *Journal of Evaluation in Clinical Practice*, 26(6), 1629–1637.

Hossain, M.Z et al. (2020). Awareness and understanding of dementia in South Asians: A synthesis of qualitative evidence. *Dementia*, 19(5), 1441–1473.

Hyatt, R. (2019). Why more South Asian families are caring for dying loved ones at home. BirminghamLive. Retrieved 14 October 2024 from: www.birminghammail.co.uk/black-country/more-south-asian-families-caring-17045568

Ige-Elegbede, J. et al. (2019). Barriers and facilitators of physical activity among adults and older adults from Black and Minority Ethnic groups in the UK: A systematic review of qualitative studies. *Preventive Medicine Reports*, 15, 100952.

Islam, Z., Taylor, L. & Faull, C. (2021). Thinking ahead in advanced illness: Exploring clinicians' perspectives on discussing resuscitation with patients and families from ethnic minority communities. *Future Healthcare Journal*, 8(3), e619–e624.

Jerwood, J. & Allen, G. (2023). *No Barriers Here: For people excluded by identity, culture, ethnicity and race*. Stourbridge: The Mary Stevens Hospice.

Johl, N. et al. (2016). What do we know about the attitudes, experiences and needs of Black and minority ethnic carers of people with dementia in the United Kingdom? A systematic review. *Dementia*, 15(4), 721–742.

Johnson, K.S. (2013). Racial and ethnic disparities in palliative care. *Journal of Palliative Medicine*, 16(11), 1329–1334.

Jong, J. et al. (2017). The religious correlates of death anxiety: A systematic review and meta-analysis. *Religion, Brain & Behavior*, 8(1), 4–20.

Kagawa-Singer, M. & Blackhall, L.J. (2001). Negotiating cross-cultural issues at the end of life: 'You got to go where he lives'. *JAMA*, 286(23), 2993–3001.

Kenning, C. et al. (2017). Barriers and facilitators in accessing dementia care by ethnic minority groups: A meta-synthesis of qualitative studies. *BMC Psychiatry*, 17(1), 316.

Khan, F. & Tadros, G. (2014). Complexity in cognitive assessment of elderly British minority ethnic groups: Cultural perspective. *Dementia (London)*, 13(4), 467–482.

Khan, G., Mirza, N. & Waheed, W. (2022). Developing guidelines for the translation and cultural adaptation of the Montreal Cognitive Assessment: Scoping review and qualitative synthesis. *BJPsych Open*, 8(1), e21.

Kim, J.H., Knight, B.G. & Longmire, C.V. (2007). The role of familism in stress and coping processes among African American and White dementia caregivers: Effects on mental and physical health. *Health Psychology*, 26(5), 564–576.

Klass, D., Silverman, P.R. & Nickman, S. (2014). *Continuing Bonds: New Understandings of Grief*. New York: Routledge.

Koch, T. & Iliffe, S. (2010). EVIDEM-ED project. Rapid appraisal of barriers to the diagnosis and management of patients with dementia in primary care: A systematic review. *BMC Family Practice*, 11, 52.

Koffman, J. (2018). *Dementia and end of life care for black, Asian and minority ethnic communities*. Better Health Briefing 45. London: Race Equality Foundation.

Kuslansky, G. et al. (2002). Screening for Alzheimer's disease: The memory impairment screen versus the conventional three-word memory test. *Journal of the American Geriatric Society*, 50(6), 1086–1091.

La Fontaine, J. et al. (2007). Understanding dementia amongst people in minority ethnic and cultural groups. *Journal of Advanced Nursing*, 60(6), 605–614.

Lam, J. et al. (2023). How is ethnicity reported, described, and analysed in health research in the UK? A bibliographical review and focus group discussions with young refugees. *BMC Public Health*, 23(1), 2025.

Leadership Alliance for the Care of Dying People (2014). *One chance to get it right: Improving people's experience of care in the last few days and hours of life*. https://assets.publishing.service.gov.uk/media/5a7e301ced915d74e33f09ee/One_chance_to_get_it_right.pdf

Leventhal, H., Phillips, L.A. & Burns, E. (2016). The Common-Sense Model of Self-Regulation (CSM): A dynamic framework for understanding illness self-management. *Journal of Behavioral Medicine*, 39(6), 935–946.

Lewis, C. & Cotterell, N. (2017). *Social isolation and older black, Asian and minority ethnic people in Greater Manchester. A report for ambition for ageing*. www.ambitionforageing.org.uk/social-isolation-and-older-black-asian-and-minority-ethnic-people-greater-manchester.

Lievesley, N. (2013). *The ageing of the ethnic minority populations of England and Wales: Findings from the 2011 census*. Centre for Policy on Ageing.

Lindeza, P. et al. (2020). Impact of dementia on informal care: A systematic review of family caregivers' perceptions. *BMJ Supportive & Palliative Care*. doi: 10.1136/bmjspcare-2020-002242

REFERENCES

Livingston, G. *et al.* (2017). Dementia prevention, intervention, and care. *The Lancet*, 390(10113), 2673–2734.

Livingston, G. *et al.* (2020). Dementia prevention, intervention, and care: 2020 report of the Lancet Commission. *The Lancet*, 396(10248), 413–446.

Lu, C. *et al.* (2022). Use of race, ethnicity, and ancestry data in health research. *PLOS Global Public Health*, 2(9), e0001060.

Lyonette, C. & Yardley, L. (2003). The influence on carer wellbeing of motivations to care for older people and the relationship with the care recipient. *Ageing & Society*, 23(4), 487–506.

Malek-Ahmadi, M. *et al.* (2012). Validation and diagnostic accuracy of the Alzheimer's questionnaire. *Age and Ageing*, 41(3), 396–399.

Mansour, R. *et al.* (2020). Late-life depression in people from ethnic minority backgrounds: Differences in presentation and management. *Journal of Affective Disorders*, 264, 340–347.

Manzoor, S. (2011). Asian parents in care homes. *The Guardian*. www.theguardian.com/lifeandstyle/2011/feb/26/asian-parents-care-homes-sarfraz-manzoor

Manthorpe, J. *et al.* (2010). *Supporting black and minority ethnic older people's mental wellbeing: Accounts of social care practice. Project report.* Social Care Instutute for Excellence. https://kar.kent.ac.uk/68379

Manthorpe, J. *et al.* (2018). Workforce diversity and conflicts in care work: Managers' perspectives. *International Journal of Care and Caring*, 2(4), 499–513.

Marie Curie. (2014). *Next steps: Improving end of life care for Black, Asian and Minority Ethnic people in the UK*. Retrieved 16 October 2024 from: www.mariecurie.org.uk/document/improving-end-of-life-care-for-minority-ethnics-in-the-uk

Mawaka, T.P. (2018). *Exploring the lived experience of the individual of Black ethnicity living with dementia: A phenomenological study.* Prof doc thesis, London South Bank University School of Health and Social Care. https://doi.org/10.18744/PUB.002090

Michie, S. *et al.* (2005). Making psychological theory useful for implementing evidence based practice: A consensus approach. *Quality and Safety in Health Care*, 14(1), 26–33.

Michie, S., van Stralen, M.M. & West, R. (2011). The behaviour change wheel: A new method for characterising and designing behaviour change interventions. *Implementation Science*, 6, 42.

Milne, A. & Smith, J. (2015). Dementia, Ethnicity and Care Homes. In J. Botsford & K. Harrison Dening (eds), *Dementia, Culture and Ethnicity: Issues for All* (197–218). London: Jessica Kingsley Publishers.

Mir, G. *et al.* (2019). Delivering a culturally adapted therapy for Muslim clients with depression. *Cognitive Behaviour Therapist*, 12, e26. doi:10.1017/S1754470X19000059

Mirza, N., Panagioti, M. & Waheed, W. (2018). Cultural validation of the Addenbrooke's Cognitive Examination Version III Urdu for the British Urdu-speaking population: A qualitative assessment using cognitive interviewing. *BMJ Open*, 8(12), e021057. doi: 10.1136/bmjopen-2017-021057

Mitchell, G. *et al.* (2017). Evaluation of 'Dementia Friends' programme for undergraduate nursing students: Innovative practice. *Dementia (London)*, 16(8), 1075–1080.

Mold, F., Fitzpatrick, J.M. & Roberts, J.D. (2005). Minority ethnic elders in care homes: A review of the literature. *Age and Ageing*, 34(2), 107–113.

Moore, V. & Cahill, S. (2013). Diagnosis and disclosure of dementia: A comparative qualitative study of Irish and Swedish general practitioners. *Aging & Mental Health*, 17(1), 77–84.

Morrish, J. et al. (2022). Group experiences of cognitive stimulation therapy (CST) in Tanzania: A qualitative study. *Aging & Mental Health*, 26(4), 688–697.

Mosdøl, A. et al. (2017). Targeted mass media interventions promoting healthy behaviours to reduce risk of non-communicable diseases in adult, ethnic minorities. *Cochrane Database of Systemic Reviews*, 2(2), CD011683.

Mountford, W. & Dening, K.H. (2019). Considering culture and ethnicity in family-centred dementia care at the end of life: A case study. *International Journal of Palliative Nursing*, 25(2), 56–64.

Mountford, W., Dening, K.H. & Green, J. (2024). Advance care planning and decision-making in dementia care: a literature review. *Nursing Older People*, doi: 10.7748/nop.2020.e1238

Mukadam, N., Cooper, C. & Livingston, G. (2013). Improving access to dementia services for people from minority ethnic groups. *Current Opinion in Psychiatry*, 26(4), 409–414.

Mukadam, N., Cooper, C. & Livingston, G. (2018). The EAST-Dem study: A pilot cluster randomized controlled trial. *International Psychogeriatrics*, 30(5), 769–773.

Mukadam, N. et al. (2011). Why do ethnic elders present later to UK dementia services? A qualitative study. *International Psychogeriatrics*, 23(7), 1070–1077.

Mukadam, N. et al. (2015). What would encourage help-seeking for memory problems among UK-based South Asians? A qualitative study. *BMJ Open*, 5(9), e007990.

Mukadam, N. et al. (2019). Ethnic differences in cognition and age in people diagnosed with dementia: A study of electronic health records in two large mental healthcare providers. *International Journal of Geriatric Psychiatry*, 34(3), 504–510.

Mukadam, N. et al. (2020). Effective interventions for potentially modifiable risk factors for late-onset dementia: A costs and cost-effectiveness modelling study. *Lancet Healthy Longevity*, 1(1), e13–e20.

Mukadam, N. et al. (2022). Risk factors, ethnicity and dementia: A UK Biobank prospective cohort study of White, South Asian and Black participants. *PLoS One*, 17(10), e0275309.

Nasreddine, Z.S. et al. (2005). The Montreal Cognitive Assessment, MoCA: A brief screening tool for mild cognitive impairment [published correction appears in the *Journal of the American Geriatric Society* (2019) 67(9), 1991]. *Journal of the American Geriatric Society*, 53(4), 695–699.

National Council for Palliative Care and National End of Life Care Programme. (2013). *Advance decisions to refuse treatment: A guide for health and social care professionals*. Retrieved 14 October 2024 from: www.england.nhs.uk/improvement-hub/wp-content/uploads/sites/44/2017/11/Advance-Decisions-to-Refuse-Treatment-Guide.pdf

National Health Service. (2024). Primary care dementia data, August 2024. Retrieved 15 October 2024 from: https://digital.nhs.uk/data-and-information/publications/statistical/primary-care-dementia-data/august-2024

National Institute for Health and Care Excellence. (2018). *Dementia: Assessment, management and support for people living with dementia and their carers*. NICE guideline [NG97]. Retrieved 11 October 2024 from: www.nice.org.uk/guidance/ng97

National Institute for Health and Care Excellence. (2021, updated 2023). *Tobacco: Preventing uptake, promoting quitting and treating dependence*. [NG209]. Retrieved 11 October 2024 from: www.nice.org.uk/guidance/ng209

REFERENCES

National Institute for Health and Care Excellence. (2024). NICE and health inequalities. Retrieved 11 October 2024 from: www.nice.org.uk/about/what-we-do/nice-and-health-inequalities

National Palliative and End of Life Care Partnership. (2021). *Ambitions for palliative and end of life care: A national framework for local action 2021–2026*. Retrieved 16 October 2024 from: www.england.nhs.uk/publication/ambitions-for-palliative-and-end-of-life-care-a-national-framework-for-local-action-2021-2026

Newbronner, L. et al. (2013). *A road less rocky – supporting carers of people with dementia*. London: Carers' Trust. Retrieved 12 October 2024 from https://carers.org/resources/all-resources/84-a-road-less-rocky-a-supporting-carers-of-people-with-dementia

NHS England. (2022) *Palliative and end of life care: Statutory guidance for integrated care boards (ICBs)*. PR1673. Retrieved 14 October 2024 from: www.england.nhs.uk/wp-content/uploads/2022/07/Palliative-and-End-of-Life-Care-Statutory-Guidance-for-Integrated-Care-Boards-ICBs-September-2022.pdf

Nielsen, T.R. & Jørgensen, K. (2020). Cross-cultural dementia screening using the Rowland Universal Dementia Assessment Scale: A systematic review and meta-analysis. *International Psychogeriatrics*, 32(9), 1031–1044.

Office for National Statistics. (2023). *Profile of the older population living in England and Wales in 2021 and changes since 2011*. Retrieved 20 October 2024 from: www.ons.gov.uk/peoplepopulationandcommunity/birthsdeathsandmarriages/ageing/articles/profileoftheolderpopulationlivinginenglandandwalesin2021andchangessince2011/2023-04-03#ethnic-group

Office for National Statistics. (2024). Cigarette smoking among adults. Retrieved 11 October 2024 from: www.ethnicity-facts-figures.service.gov.uk/health/alcohol-smoking-and-drug-use/adult-smokers/latest

Oldroyd, J. et al. (2005). Diabetes and ethnic minorities. *Postgraduate Medical Journal*, 81(958), 486–490.

Ott, C.H, Sanders, S. & Kelber, S.T. (2007). Grief and personal growth experience of spouses and adult-child caregivers of persons with Alzheimer's disease or related dementias. *The Gerontologist*, 47, 798–809.

Owen, J.E., Goode, K.T. & Haley, W.E. (2001). End of life care and reactions to death in African-American and white family caregivers of relatives with Alzheimer's disease. *Omega (Westport)*, 43(4), 349–361.

Parveen, S., Blakey, H. & Oyebode, J.R. (2018). Evaluation of a carers' information programme culturally adapted for South Asian families. *International Journal of Geriatric Psychiatry*, 33(2), e199–e204.

Parveen, S., Barker, S., Kaur, R., Kerry, F., Mitchell, W., Happs, A., Fry, G., Morrison, V., Fortinsky, R. and Oyebode, J.R., 2018. Involving minority ethnic communities and diverse experts by experience in dementia research: the caregiving HOPE study. *Dementia*, 17(8), 990 -1000.

Parveen, S, Morrison, V. & Robinson, C.A. (2011). Ethnic variations in the caregiver role: A qualitative study. *Journal of Health Psychology*, 16(6), 862–872.

Parveen, S., Morrison, V. & Robinson, C.A. (2013). Ethnicity, familism and willingness to care: Important influences on caregiver mood? *Aging & Mental Health*, 17(1), 115–124.

Parveen, S., Peltier, C. & Oyebode, J.R. (2017). Perceptions of dementia and use of services in minority ethnic communities: A scoping exercise. *Health & Social Care Community*, 25(2), 734–742.

Patel, N. et al. (2017). Barriers and facilitators to healthy lifestyle changes in minority ethnic populations in the UK: A narrative review. *Journal of Racial & Ethnic Health Disparities*, 4(6), 1107–1119.

Pham, T.M. et al. (2018). Trends in dementia diagnosis rates in UK ethnic groups: Analysis of UK primary care data. *Clinical Epidemiology*, 10, 949–960.

Phipps, E. et al. (2003). Approaching the end of life: Attitudes, preferences, and behaviors of African-American and white patients and their family caregivers. *Journal of Clinical Oncology*, 21(3), 549–554.

Poole, C., Harrison, J. & Hill, J. (2021). Understanding dementia in South Asian populations: An exploration of knowledge and awareness. *British Journal of Neuroscience Nursing*, 17(4), 56–159.

Poscia, A. et al. (2018). Interventions targeting loneliness and social isolation among the older people: An update systematic review. *Experimental Gerontology*, 102, 133–144.

Prajapati, R. & Liebling, H. (2022). Accessing mental health services: A systematic review and meta-ethnography of the experiences of South Asian service users in the UK. *Journal of Racial and Ethnic Health Disparities*, 9(2), 598–619.

Prince, M. et al. (2014) *Dementia UK: Update*. Second edition. King's College London, https://www.alzheimers.org.uk/sites/default/files/migrate/downloads/dementia_uk_update.pdf

Prince, M. et al. (2015) *World Alzheimer Report 2015. The global impact of dementia: An analysis of prevalence, incidence, cost and trends*. Alzheimer's Disease International, https://www.alzint.org/u/WorldAlzheimerReport2015.pdf

Public Health England. (2016). *Faith at end of life: A resource for professionals, providers and commissioners working in communities*. Retrieved 14 October 2024 from: www.gov.uk/government/publications/faith-at-end-of-life-public-health-approach-resource-for-professionals

Quinn, C. et al. (2022). Living well with dementia: What is possible and how to promote it. *International Journal of Geriatric Psychiatry*, 37(1), 10.1002/gps.5627

Rathod, S. et al. (2018). The current status of culturally adapted mental health interventions: A practice-focused review of meta-analyses. *Neuropsychiatric Disease and Treatment*, 14, 165–178.

Rauf, M.A. (2023). Optimisation of care transitions: Understanding coping *strategies of South Asian family carers of a relative with advanced dementia*. https://bradscholars.brad.ac.uk/entities/publication/0ab00316-4e10-4100-bb8d-ceef3debcc19

Regan, J.L. et al. (2013). A systematic review of religion and dementia care pathways in black and minority ethnic populations. *Mental Health, Religion & Culture*, 16(1), 1–15.

Riley, G.A., Evans, L. & Oyebode, J.R. (2018). Relationship continuity and emotional well-being in spouses of people with dementia. *Aging & Mental Health*, 22(3), 299–305.

Roche, M. et al. (2018). The IDEMCare Study – Improving Dementia Care in Black African and Caribbean Groups: A feasibility cluster randomised controlled trial. *International Journal of Geriatric Psychiatry*, 33(8), 1048–1056.

Roche, M. et al. (2021). A review of qualitative research of perception and experiences of dementia among adults from Black, African, and Caribbean background: What and whom are we researching? *Gerontologist*, 61(5), e195–e208.

Rowland, J.T. et al. (2006). The Rowland Universal Dementia Assessment Scale (RUDAS) and the Folstein MMSE in a multicultural cohort of elderly persons. *International Psychogeriatrics*, 18(1), 111–120.

REFERENCES

Ryder, M. *et al.* (2021). BAME: A report on the use of the term and responses to it: Terminology review for the BBC and creative industries. www.open-access.bcu.ac.uk/14959

Sampson, E. L., White, N., Lord, K., Leurent, B., Vickerstaff, V., & Jones, L. (2006). Differences in prescribing for dementia patients from ethnic minorities: A review of health inequalities in dementia care. *Aging & Mental Health*, 10(3), 221–228. https://doi.org/10.1080/13607860500310504

Sayegh, P. & Knight, B.G. (2013). Cross-cultural differences in dementia: The Sociocultural Health Belief Model. *International Psychogeriatrics*, 25(4), 517–530.

Shafiq, S. (2024). *Using the self-regulatory model to explore cultural understandings of dementia and inform a culturally sensitive intervention.* https://bradscholars.brad.ac.uk/entities/publication/963b56e5-f8c1-4d4a-ab35-c6123b612e15

Shankley, W., Hannemann, T. & Simpson, L. (2020). The Demography of Ethnic Minorities in Britain. In B. Byrne, C. Alexander, O. Khan, J. Nazroo & W. Shankley (eds), *Ethnicity, Race and Inequality in the UK: State of the Nation* (pp.15–34). Bristol: Policy Press.

Shannon, K., Bail, K. & Neville, S. (2019). Dementia-friendly community initiatives: An integrative review. *Journal of Clinical Nursing*, 28(11–12), 2035–2045.

Shaw, A.R. *et al.* (2022). Representation of racial and ethnic minority populations in dementia prevention trials: A systematic review. *Journal of Prevention of Alzheimer's Disease*, 9(1), 113–118.

Shiekh, S.I. *et al.* (2021). Ethnic differences in dementia risk: A systematic review and meta-analysis. *Journal of Alzheimer's Disease*, 80(1), 337–355.

Skills for Health. (2018). *Dementia Training Standards Framework.* www.skillsforhealth.org.uk/wp-content/uploads/2021/01/Dementia-Core-Skills-Education-and-Training-Framework.pdf

Spector, A. *et al.* (2019). Mixed methods implementation research of cognitive stimulation therapy (CST) for dementia in low and middle-income countries: Study protocol for Brazil, India and Tanzania (CST-International). *BMJ Open*, 9(8), e030933.

Stroebe, M. & Schut, H. (1999). The dual process model of coping with bereavement: Rationale and description. *Death Studies*, 23: 197–224.

Todd, S. *et al.* (2013). Survival in dementia and predictors of mortality: A review. *International Journal of Geriatric Psychiatry*, 28(11), 1109–1124.

Tsamakis, K. *et al.* (2021). Dementia in people from ethnic minority backgrounds: Disability, functioning, and pharmacotherapy at the time of diagnosis. *Journal of the American Medical Directors Association*, 22(2), 446–452.

Tuerk, R. & Sauer, J. (2015). Dementia in a Black and minority ethnic population: Characteristics of presentation to an inner London memory service. *BJPsych Bulletin*, 39(4), 162–166.

UK Government. (2024). *Ethnic groups by household type.* Retrieved 15 October 2024 from: www.ethnicity-facts-figures.service.gov.uk/uk-population-byethnicity/demographics/families-and-households/latest

Valtorta, N.K. *et al.* (2018). Loneliness, social isolation and risk of cardiovascular disease in the English Longitudinal Study of Ageing. *European Journal of Preventive Cardiology*, 25(13), 1387–1396.

Victor, C.R. *et al.* (2024). Living well with dementia: An exploratory matched analysis of minority ethnic and white people with dementia and carers participating in the IDEAL programme. *International Journal of Geriatric Psychiatry*, 39(1), e6048.

Waheed, W. *et al.* (2020). Developing and implementing guidelines on culturally adapting the Addenbrooke's cognitive examination version III (ACE-III): A qualitative illustration. *BMC Psychiatry*, 20(1), 492.

Ward, C. (2008). Thinking outside the Berry boxes: New perspectives on identity, acculturation and intercultural relations. *International Journal of Intercultural Relations*, 32(2), 105–114.

Weinman, J. *et al.* (1996). The illness perception questionnaire: A new method for assessing the cognitive representation of illness. *Psychology & Health*, 11(3), 431–445.

Wilkinson, E. *et al.* (2016). Meeting the challenge of diabetes in ageing and diverse populations: A review of the literature from the UK. *Journal of Diabetes Research*, 8030627.

Williams, E.D. *et al.* (2015). Depressive symptoms are doubled in older British South Asian and Black Caribbean people compared with Europeans: Associations with excess co-morbidity and socioeconomic disadvantage. *Psychological Medicine*, 45(9), 1861–1871.

Wilson, A. *et al.* (2020). Ethnic variations in referrals to the Leicester memory and dementia assessment service, 2010 to 2017. *BJPsych Open*, 6(5), e83.

Wittenberg, R. *et al.* (2019). The costs of dementia in England. *International Journal of Geriatric Psychiatry*, 34(7), 1095–1103.

World Health Organization. (2024a). *WHO global report on trends in prevalence of tobacco use 2000–2030*. World Health Organization.

World Health Organization. (2024b). Social determinants of health. Retrieved 11 October 2024 from: www.who.int/health-topics/social-determinants-of-health#tab=tab_1

Wright, A.A. *et al.* (2008). Associations between end-of-life discussions, patient mental health, medical care near death, and caregiver bereavement adjustment. *JAMA*, 300(14), 1665–1673.

Youn, G. *et al.* (1999). Differences in familism values and caregiving outcomes among Korean, Korean American, and White American dementia caregivers. *Psychology and Aging*, 14(3), 355–364.

Subject Index

Sub-headings in *italics* indicate figures and tables.

abusive situations 98–100
acculturation 43, 101
activities 14
   design a dementia
      awareness information
      programme for the
      Nigerian community
      living in the UK 55
   design your own social
      media campaign 35–6
   How are you? quiz 16
   identifying and acting
      on culturally related
      issues 117–18, 120
   identifying culturally suitable
      activities 111–12
   identifying risk factors from
      case studies 27–9
   knowing the facts of
      assessment and
      diagnosis for minority
      ethnic groups 61–2
   living well with dementia 88–9
   motivations for care 84–5, 95
   preparing for transition
      points 87
   using the Common Sense
      model to think about
      dementia 46–7
   what do you think of when you
      think of dementia? 37
   your plan for improving access
      to dementia assessment
      for people from minority
      ethnic communities 67
ADAPT study 49–50, 53, 70, 73, 75, 76, 90
Addenbrooke's Cognitive
   Examination (ACE) 73, 75, 149
   ACE-III 74
advance care planning 124, 151–2
   addressing advance care
      planning with people
      from minority ethnic
      communities 128
   advance decision to refuse
      treatment (ADRT) 124
   advance statements 124
   barriers to advance care
      planning 126–7
   do not resuscitate orders
      (DNRs) 124
   NHS websites 124
   No Barriers Here© 128–9
   why do advance care
      planning? 125
alcohol consumption 20
Alzheimer's Questionnaire 76
Alzheimer's Research UK 80
Alzheimer's Society 38, 47–8, 66, 69, 72
   Information Programme
      for South Asian
      Families (IPSAF) 7, 51
anticipatory grief 140

Assessment of Motor and
    Process Skills (AMPS) 75

barriers to advance care
    planning 126
  cultural values 126
  delayed diagnosis 126
  distrust of services 127
  lack of dementia awareness
    126
  legal frameworks 127
  religious beliefs 126–7
  staff assumptions 127
barriers to diagnosis 62
  community barriers to seeking
    assessment 62–4
  service barriers to
    assessment 65
  ways forward 65–7
behaviour change 30
  *Barriers to behavioural
    change* 31
  evaluation and monitoring 33
  identify barriers to behaviour
    change 31–2
  identify behaviour to be
    changed 30–1
  matching barriers to behaviour
    change techniques 32
  *Matching behaviour change
    techniques to barriers*
    154–5
  principles of effective health
    communication 33–6
  *Strategies to overcome
    barriers* 32
bereavement 139, 152–3
  post-death factors
    affecting adjustment to
    bereavement 141–3
  pre-death factors affecting
    caregiver grief 139–41
Bradford 41, 140–1
brain health 8, 10, 18, 41, 48, 89, 147
  brain scans 68
  traumatic brain injuries 20

care homes 97–8, 119–20, 150–1
  deciding whether to use a
    care home 98–106
  living in a care home 106–19
care in the community
    79, 94–5, 149–50
  access to support 90–2
  caregiving and family
    dynamics 80–1
  cultural and religious
    influences on
    family care 81–4
  cultural competence for
    practitioners 92–4
  living well with dementia 87–90
  motivations, willingness and
    preparedness to care 84–7
  who is the carer? 80–1
Caregiving HOPE study 7, 48, 79,
    80–2, 85–6, 97, 101–5, 119
Carers Trust 87
Centre for Applied Dementia
    Studies, University of
    Bradford 8, 116, 117
Chadha, Divya 9, 99, 101, 102
Cheston, Richard 8
cognitive assessments 71–2
  *Barriers to the validity of
    cognitive assessments
    for minority ethnic
    populations* 71–2
  cognitive assessment in
    dementia assessment
    services 73–5
  cognitive screening in
    primary care 72–3
cognitive stimulation therapy 90
Common Sense model
    of illness 44–7
Covid-19 pandemic 39
cultural and religious influences
    on family care 81–4
cultural perspectives on
    dementia 40–1
  religion 41–2
culturally competent engagement
    with communities 52–5

SUBJECT INDEX

A checklist for cultural adaptation of dementia awareness materials 53–5
cultural competence for practitioners 92–4
interviewing and history-taking 69–71
Ten top tips for your cultural competency learning journey 94

deciding whether to use a care home 98, 119–20
abusive situations 98–100
coping with stigma 103–5
different family configurations 105–6
Examples of external pressures to continue to care at home 103
societal and generational changes 103
DEM-SAFE project 8
dementia 9, 14, 145–53
dementia and ethnicity 10–11
see risk factors
dementia as a terminal illness 122–3, 143–4, 151
advance care planning 124–9
being bereaved of a relative with dementia 139–43
palliative and end-of-life care 123, 129–38
'service gap' in palliative and end-of-life care 130
dementia assessment 57–8, 67–8, 77
A model for interventions to improve access to dementia assessment and services for people from ethnic minorities 66
cognitive assessment in dementia assessment services 73–5
cognitive screening and assessment 71–2

cognitive screening in primary care 72–3
community barriers to seeking assessment 62–4
functional assessment 75
interviewing and history-taking 69–71
knowing the facts of assessment and diagnosis for minority ethnic groups 61–2
language and interpretation 68–9
minority ethnic referrals for dementia assessment 58–9
service barriers to assessment 65
speaking with family members 76–7
dementia awareness 37, 55–6, 145
Common Sense model of illness 45–6
cultural perspectives on dementia 40–3
importance of dementia awareness 38
Key factors that influence perceptions of illness 44
promoting dementia awareness and education 47–52
understanding perceptions of dementia 44–7
using the Common Sense model to think about dementia 46–7
Dementia Friends 38–9, 47–8
Dementia Training Standards Framework 93
Department of Health 93
depression 19, 23–4
diabetes 19, 21–2, 66
diagnosis 38–9, 57–8, 77, 148–9
are people from minority ethnic backgrounds more or less likely to be diagnosed with dementia? 60
background statistics 58–62

diagnosis *cont.*
  barriers to diagnosis 62–7
  dementia assessment 67–77
  do people from minority ethnic backgrounds approach services later? 59
  do people from minority ethnic backgrounds get dementia earlier in life? 60–1
  knowing the facts of assessment and diagnosis for minority ethnic groups 61–2
dying 135
  clinical practice 135–6
  faith, religion and spirituality 136–7
  Key recommendations for health and care professionals formulating end-of-live care plans for people from ethnic minorities 138
  preferred place of death 136

East-Dem project 51
education 18
end-of-life care 121, 143–4, 152
  advance care planning 124–9
  bereavement 139–43
  definitions, facts and figures 122–3
  end of life care 129–38
  see palliative care
ethnicity 9, 119
  dementia and ethnicity 10–11
  ethnic minorities in the UK 13–14
  terminology 11–12

familism 82, 83, 103
family members 76–7
  cultural and religious influences on family care 81–4
  importance of working with families 103
  post-death factors affecting adjustment to bereavement 141–3
  pre-death factors affecting caregiver grief 139–41
  preparing for transition points in dementia caregiving 87
functional assessment 75

GPs 51, 59, 65, 68, 77, 90, 137, 148–9
grief 139
  anticipatory grief 140
  chronic sorrow 139–40
  consequences of caregiving 140–1
Guardian, The 113

health 26
  Five layers of health determinants 27
  health inequities and health inequalities 26–7, 145–6
  health communication 33–4
  designing a social media campaign 35–6
  Top ten points for designing effective mass media health campaigns 34–5
Health Education England 93
hearing loss 18
heart disease 19, 21, 24, 766
history-taking 69–71
  speaking with family members 76–7
hypertension 19, 21–2

IDEMcare project 51
interviews 69–71

Jewish Care 107

language and interpretation 68–9, 113
  Approaches to improving communication between staff and care home residents who do not speak fluent English 114

SUBJECT INDEX

translating 'dementia' into
'memory problems' 49, 147
lifestyles 15, 146–7
  achieving behaviour
    change 30–3
  ethnic differences in
    dementia risk 16–17
  identifying risk factors 27–30
  modifiable risk factors 17–20
  modifiable risk factors
    and minority ethnic
    communities 20–6
living in a care home 106
  culturally specific care
    homes 107
  numbers of people from
    minority ethnic
    communities living in
    care homes 106–7
living in a 'generic' care
  home 108, 117–18
  communication 112–14
  diversity among staff 118
  faith and religion 114–16
  food 109–10
  personal care 108–9
  racism 116–17
  social connection and
    activities 110–12
  steps towards culturally
    appropriate care
    for minority ethnic
    residents 118–19
living well with dementia 87–90

majority ethnic communities 13
  dementia and stigma 39
Marie Curie 133
Memory Impairment Screen 73
Mini Mental State Examination
  (MMSE) 59
Mini-Cog 73
minority ethnic communities
  13–14, 145–53
  access to support in
    dementia care 90–2
  comparisons in dementia
    diagnoses with people
      from majority ethnic
      backgrounds 59–61
  cultural perspectives on
    dementia 40–3, 147
  culturally competent
    engagement with
    communities 52–5
  culturally competent
    engagement with
    communities 52–5
  dementia awareness 37–9,
    55–6
  improving minority ethnic
    communities' experience
    of palliative care 133–8
  minority ethnic referrals for
    dementia assessment 58–9
  modifiable risk factors of
    dementia 20–6, 36
  palliative and end-of-life care
    for dementia 130–3
  promoting dementia awareness
    and education 47–52
  promoting dementia awareness
    and education 47–52
  societal and generational
    changes 100–3
  understanding perceptions
    of dementia 44–7
Montreal Cognitive Assessment
  (MoCA) 73, 74, 75, 149
motivations for caregiving 84–7
  preparing for transition points
    in dementia caregiving 87
mourning 141–2
  continuing bonds after
    death 142
  mourning rituals 142–3
  religious faith 142

National Institute for Health and
  Care Research (NIHR) 8
No Barriers Here© 128–9

obesity 19, 21–2

palliative care 123, 129–30, 143–4, 152
   access to care 131
   clinical practice 135–6
   Domains of the culturagram assessment framework 135–6
   faith, religion and spirituality 136–8
   general frameworks and guidance 134–5
   improving minority ethnic communities' experience of palliative care 133–8
   Key recommendations for health and care professionals formulating end-of-live care plans for people from ethnic minorities 138
   minority ethnic people with dementia 130–3
   preferred place of death 136
   quality of care 131–2
   reasons for poor experiences 132–3
   service support 133–4
physical activity 18, 21–2
points for practice 14
   ADAPT toolkit 50
   ask about mourning rituals 142–3
   ask about support networks 106
   be respectfully curious about religion 116
   co-develop ethnically appropriate care plans 138
   communication needs 113–14
   consider safeguarding issues 100
   dementia assessment tests for the South Asian communities 75
   early signs of cognitive impairment in ethnic minority groups 71
   getting personal care right 109
   greetings 70
   identifying the carers 81
   importance of working with families 103
   inclusive community services 92
   individual food preferences 109
   keeping ethnicity on the agenda 119
   limitations of brief cognitive screening tests 73
   offer a follow-up appointment after bereavement 141
   staff who speak different languages 68
   support family members to adjust if a relative moves to a care home 105
   taking a history 77
   use creative approaches to enable conversations about future care 129
   using the assessment of motor and process skills 75
points for reflection 14
   changes in motivations for caregiving over time 86
   translating 'dementia' into 'memory problems' 49
   ensure people are well-informed about end-of-life care 134
power of attorney 125, 127

Race Equality Foundation 128, 130
racism 24, 25, 70, 97, 106, 108, 116–17, 151
religion 41–2, 63
   care homes 114–16
   church leaders 90
   cultural and religious influences on family care 81–4
   end of life planning 126–7
   imams 104–5
   mourning rituals 142–3
risk factors 15, 36
   broader context of health 26–7

dementia and modifiable
    risk factors 17–20
ethnic differences in
    dementia risk 16–17
lifestyle changes to delay the
    onset of dementia 27–33
modifiable risk factors
    and minority ethnic
    communities 20–6
principles of effective health
    communication 33–6
Rowland Universal Dementia
    Assessment Scale
    (RUDAS) 74, 75, 149

safeguarding issues 100
Six Item Cognitive Impairment
    Test (6-CIT) 71–2
smoking 19, 22–3
Social Care Institute for
    Excellence (SCIE) 130
social contact 19, 24–6
sorrow 139, 40
stigma 37, 55–6, 103–5, 147
    cultural perspectives on
        dementia 40–3

culturally competent
    engagement with
    communities 52–5
importance of dementia
    awareness 38–9
promoting dementia awareness
    and education 47–52
understanding perceptions
    of dementia 44–7

Theoretical Domains Framework
    (TDF) 30–1, 146

UK National Dementia
    Strategy 38
University of Bradford 7, 93, 117

vascular dementia 60

World Alzheimer Report 17

xiao (filial piety) 82–3

Author Index

Action on Smoking and Health 23
Adelman, S. 59
Age UK. 25
Akarsu, N.E. 90
All Party Parliamentary Group on Dementia (APPG) 13
Allen, G. 129
Alzheimer's Disease International 38
Alzheimer's Research UK 80
Alzheimer's Society 66, 73, 109
Arblaster, K. 66
Aspinall, P.J. 11

Badger, F. 106, 108, 109, 112, 114, 115, 118
Bail, K. 48
Baillie, L. 48
Banerjee, S. 105
Beecraft, S. 48
Berning, M.J. 48
Berwald, S. 37, 62
Bifarin, O.O. 7, 183
Birch, D. 130
Blackhall, L.J. 126
Blakemore, A. 63, 64
Blakey, H. 7, 51, 140–1
Bothongo, P.L. 16
Brayne, C. 123
Brodaty, H. 122
Brottman, M.R. 93
Burns, E. 45
Buschke, H. 73

Cahill, K.M. 83
Cahill, S. 65
Calanzani, N. 131, 133
Capstick, A. 117
Care Act 2014 100
Care Quality Commission (CQC) 133
Carers UK 91
Chan, D. 140, 142
Co, M. 122, 123
Collins, L. 116
Cook, L. 58, 65
Cooper, C. 50, 51, 52, 65, 107, 113, 119
Cordell, C.B. 73
Cotterell, N. 24
Cova, I. 74
Cuibus, M.V. 13

Dahlgren, G. 26, 27
Dementia, UK 60
Dening, K.H. 126, 135
Department of Health and Social Care 38, 57
Devonport, T.J. 24
Dixon, J. 131, 133, 136
Dlamini, T. 126, 127
Draper, J. 130

Evans, L. 140
Evans, N. 132

Faull, C. 133
Fischer, A.G. 75
Fitzpatrick, J.M. 113, 118
Folstein, M.F. 59

AUTHOR INDEX

Folstein, S.E. 59
Fulton, R. 140

Gibson, L. 122
Giebel, C.M. 63
Goode, K.T. 140
Goodorally, V. 135
Gottesman, D.J. 140
Gove, D. 69
Green, J. 126
Griggs, J.J. 132

Hailstone, J. 64
Haley, W.E. 140
Hannemann, T. 13
Harrison, J. 40
Higginson, I. 131, 133
Hill, J. 40
Hodges, J.R. 73
Holt-Lunstad, J. 24, 25
Hoppe, S.A. 139
Hossain, M.Z. 39, 81
Hyatt, R. 121

Ige-Elegbede, J. 22
Iliffe, S. 65
Islam, Z. 133

Jerwood, J. 129
Johl, N. 39, 40, 42
Johnson, K.S. 132
Jong, J. 126
Jørgensen, K. 74

Kagawa-Singer, M. 126
Kelber, S.T. 140
Kenning, C. 50, 62, 64, 65, 66, 67
Khan, F. 64
Khan, H.T.A. 81
Khan, G. 74
Kim, J.H. 83
Klass, D. 142
Knight, B.G. 83
Koch, T. 65
Koffman, J. 130
Koffman, J. 131, 133
Kuslansky, G. 73

La Fontaine, J. 7
Lam, J. 12
Larner, A.J. 73
Leadership Alliance for the
    Care of Dying People 135
Leventhal, H. 45
Lewis, C. 24
Liebling, H. 24
Lievesley, N. 13
Lindeza, P. 80
Livingston, G. 15, 17, 18,
    20, 50, 51, 52, 65
Longmire, C.V. 83
Lu, C. 11
Lyonette, C. 84

Malek-Ahmadi, M. 76
Mansour, R. 23
Manzoor, S. 101, 113
Manthorpe, J. 107, 110, 114,
    118, 119, 130, 133
Marie Curie 134
Mawaka, T.P. 63
McHugh, P.R. 59
Michie, S. 30, 31, 32, 154
Milne, A. 107
Mir, G. 24
Mirza, N. 74
Mitchell, G. 48
Mold, F. 113, 118
Moore, V. 65
Morrish, J. 90
Morrison, V. 83
Mosdøl, A. 34
Mountford, W. 126, 135
Mukadam, N. 16, 20, 50, 51, 52,
    58, 59, 61, 62, 63, 64, 65

Nasreddine, Z.S. 73
National Council for
    Palliative Care 124
National End of Life Care
    Programme 124
National Health Service 62
National Institute for Health
    and Care Excellence
    (NICE) 23, 26, 72

National Palliative and End of
 Life Care Partnership 130
Neville, S. 48
Newbronner, L. 87
NHS England 123, 130
Nickman, S. 142
Nielsen, T.R. 74

Office for National
 Statistics 22, 131
Oldroyd, J. 21
Ott, C.H. 140
Owen, J.E. 140
Oyebode, J. 7, 39, 41, 51, 140–1

Panagioti, M. 74
Parveen, S. 7, 39, 41, 51, 83, 140–1
Patel, N. 22
Peltier, C. 7, 39, 41
Pham, T.M. 60
Phillips, L.A. 45
Phipps, E. 125, 132
Poole, C. 40
Poscia, A. 25
Prajapati, R. 24
Prince, M. 17, 106
Public Health England 136, 137–8

Quinn, C. 87, 88

Rathod, S. 24
Rauf, M.A. 7, 139, 141
Regan, J.L. 63
Riley, G.A. 140
Roberts, J.D. 113, 118
Robinson, C.A. 83
Roche, M. 40, 51, 65
Rowland, J.T. 74
Ryder, M. 11, 12

Sampson, E. L. 132
Sanders, S. 140
Sauer, J. 61
Sayegh, P. 83
Schut, H. 139
Seeher, K. 122
Shafiq, S. 7, 41, 42, 52, 57, 115, 117

Shankley, W. 13
Shannon, K. 48
Shaw, A.R. 20
Shiekh, S.I. 16
Skills for Health 93
Silverman, P.R. 142
Simpson, L. 13
Smith, J. 107
Spector, A. 90
Stroebe, M. 139

Tadros, G. 64
Taylor, L. 133
Todd, S. 10
Tsamakis, K. 60
Tuerk, R. 61

UK Government 14, 105

Valtorta, N.K. 24
van Stralen, M.M. 32
Victor, C.R. 88

Waheed, W. 74
Ward, C. 101
Weinman, J. 45
West, R. 32
Whitehead, M. 26, 27
Wilkinson, E. 21
Williams, E.D. 23
Wilson, A. 65
Wittenberg, R. 79
Woods, S. 48
World Health Organization 22, 26
Wright, A.A. 133

Yardley, L. 84
Youn, G. 83